I0425217

Let's Talk American Healthcare

How the SPUN Insurance Plan Can Solve Our Country's Medical Crisis

William Frangipane, M.D.

Copyright © 2019 William Frangipane

All rights reserved.

ISBN-13: 9781090569141

DEDICATION

To my wife, Jen, thank you for being the healer of my heart and my soul.

CONTENTS

ACKNOWLEDGMENTS

This book represents a summary of my reflections on the changes in American medicine that I observed during my career. Although our technology improved and wonder drugs appeared, the service we gave to our patients worsened. So in my retirement, I decided I would put these observations to paper. But I wanted to do more than just complain, reflect and tell old war stories. I hoped to give solutions for our expensive, ineffective, partially inclusive healthcare system. These ideas came from more than just my research. They developed from thousands of interactions with hundreds of people. I now wish to acknowledge these individuals who touched my 34 years in the medical field.

My gratitude starts with my patients who honored me by putting their trust in my medical hands. I was fortunate to work with such dedicated nurses, doctors and other health professionals. I learned hard work, empathy and teamwork from them. I had so many great teachers and mentors who became my role models. I had so many brilliant students who taught me more than I ever taught them.

But I could not have practiced medicine for even one day without the support of my family. My parents, Leo and Tina, were my first teachers. My first wife, Ann, held our family together during those endless hours when I was delivering babies. She also taught me how someone could have dignity and be selfless at the end of their life. My children, Laura and Matt, sacrificed much of their childhood for my career as I was so much only a part time parent. Finally, my second wife, Jen, taught me one can be lucky enough to fall in love twice in one lifetime.

William Frangipane, M.D.

FORWARD

Our baby was sick. Gracie, our nickname for her, Grace, did not seem herself over the past several weeks. She was not overtly ill, but as her parents, we had that uncomfortable feeling that something was not right. And at only six months of age, she could not communicate to us what was wrong. She was lethargic, not as alert as normal. She ate but less than usual and fussed at her food. There was that certain sparkle missing from her eyes. All subtle, but still worrying. As her parents, we went through both those internal and external debates about what to do. Is she okay or are we just overreacting first time parents? Should we take a wait and see approach or take her to her doctor for an evaluation?

Our dilemma of whether to take her to the doctor was more than about whether she was sick, or not. Dozens of other questions raced through our minds. Would the staff at the medical office think we were crazy? Did we want to deal with the complexity of getting her seen? You know what I mean. First, the navigation of the obnoxious phone tree, just calling the office. The rude game of ping-pong once on the phone to try to find someone, there, who would help us. The difficult car buying-like negotiations to get her an appointment. The missing of work and the complete rearrangement of the rest of our lives to get her to that appointment which, of course, would be the worst possible of times for our family. The ugly and crowded waiting room. The forms. The wait. Rude receptionists. More forms. Tattered magazines infected with the germs of the last ten sick people that came to the office. Then finally, the callback to the exam room encounter that would start the carwash-like ride that would be Gracie's appointment. Carwash? You know, being shuffled and pushed along from one place to another, being poked and prodded along the way until you arrive at the exam room. Then more waiting for the Wizard of Oz to appear.

The Wizard of Oz? Who is that, you ask? It is name for the doctor in charge of her care. The much talked about, but rarely seen power, hidden behind the magical curtain. The one you spend so much time traveling down the Yellow Brick Road and endure many detours and adventures to see. And what kind of encounter would we have with the Wizard of Oz? For in the past, the meeting with the Wizard went so many different ways. Would it be a curt and dismissive one? The two-minute encounter where you get the feeling you are wasting the almighty Wizard's time? And yours. Or the one meant to reassure you that things are normal but leaves you feeling even less comforted and more confused than when you walked in. Or would the encounter with the Wizard put you on another road trip, this time to Disney Land?

Disney Land? That is where you will be sent to a truly magical and mysterious place full of many encounters with multiple, different Wizards of Oz. Who are these other wizards? The blood tests. The x-rays. The medical specialists. Sometimes you have the fun of riding the same ride several times. And all along you are not sure if you are getting any closer to the simple answer of what the hell is the matter. Oh! When you get home from Disney Land, just like the real one, there is an unpleasant pile of expensive bills waiting for you.

What did we do in this case? We bit the bullet and made that first triggering call to Gracie's doctor. But a surprise! A real person answered the call by the second ring of the phone. Unlike other typical medical practices, they utilized that 1990s technology of caller ID and greeted us by our name. This simple gesture felt so good. How wonderful to be treated like a person, not a widget to be fitted into a hole. And they were nice! It was not like talking to the IRS or Comcast. There was no waiting on hold on the phone and being passed around to talk to three other people just to get a simple appointment. The first receptionist, the woman who answered the phone, actually was able to help us. She asked us what was wrong and within a minute offered us an appointment. There were no complex insurance questions that you do not want to deal with when you are sick or have a sick loved one. And the appointment was *that* day. It was at a time that was convenient for us. It fit our schedule, not theirs. The best was the feeling she was really trying to help us and was not just going through the motions like a dreary worker of Stalinist Russia.

When we arrived at the doctor's office, the staff was happy to see us. It was like being greeted by a family we have not seen in a while. Here was a medical staff that you could tell in an instant loved what they did for a living. They appeared to be working hard but do not seem overwhelmed. Although the office was busy, it was not chaotic, like Best Buy on Black Friday. There was no car wash ride, either. After a brief wait without time to even select a magazine or check our e-mail on our phone, we were brought back to the examination room. There was no clipboard filled with forms to fill out. You know, the same forms that you fill out every time you go to the same office with the same exact questions. No killing of trees took place for this visit that rivaled the number of legal papers for the closing of a Fortune 500 Company. No papers to explain their HIPPA privacy policy, the insurance processes or the finger wagging of how *we* could be better patients for them. The medical assistant treated us like people, not an app to be worked on, or another dreary task to be completed. Our conversation with her was…well conversational. Not an Amazon Alexa sounding, machine gun fire of questions, asked the exact same way to every patient all day long. Head cold. Brain tumor. Depression. Same questions. Same reactions. Wait! I am wrong. Alexa has more personality.

Now we are in the examination room with Gracie with that trapped, claustrophobic feeling, waiting, wondering and worrying. You know the feeling. Minutes can feel like hours in here. But as soon as we began to get that feeling, there was a knock on the door. Wonderful! No long wait to see the Wizard of Oz! And even better. From the moment the doctor entered our room, you could sense how her goal was to help Gracie, not just get us out the carwash door.

She did so in the most efficient, pleasant way possible. In medical school, they teach you that 90% of making a diagnosis is by taking a good history. Simply ask the right questions and you can find out what is wrong with almost all patients. But taking a good medical history takes time. It takes the ability to listen and to reflect and to understand and to process the information that you are getting. It also takes trust and empathy. It is a relationship, not unlike that of trying to understand what is the matter with your mate or your friend. Physicians and other healthcare providers too often shortcut this process. Because they have no time, themselves, they waste your time. Patients, instead, are sent for expensive, unnecessary, time-consuming, frightening and sometimes dangerous tests. They order everything rather than taking to the time to think. Almost as bad, they rely on a rigid protocol. Everyone with a headache gets the same, exact battery of tests. All headaches are approached in the same, exact way. Head cold. Brain tumor. Depression.

Gracie's doctor did none of these things. She asked the right questions. She pondered and responded and considered. She was kind. She smiled and built rapport with the three of us. She personalized her interview. She did not rush to judgment. A mentor of mine, a wonderful pediatric physician, Dr. Jeffery Fogel, once told me that physicians make up their minds as to a diagnosis and a treatment plan before the first thirty seconds of an encounter with a patient is over. Time constraints forces reflexive thinking. This is harmful in so many ways. Diagnoses, like mean nicknames bully dole out, stick forever. A half minute is not long enough to label anyone with anything for the rest of their lives.

Next, she examined Gracie. A real examination. She looked where it was important to look, for example spending a lot of time noting the texture of her hair. She didn't waste time doing perfunctory tasks to make it *look* like Gracie was getting an exam. You know, that two second listen to the heart and lungs that could not pick up any pathology, even if there was a cuckoo clock inside.

Finally, she gave us Gracie's diagnosis. It was a case of hypothyroidism. Gracie, she thought, had an underactive thyroid gland, causing the symptoms we were seeing. She would run a blood test to confirm the diagnosis. But it would be one test, not a shotgun approach of dozens of expensive, unrevealing and often contradictory ones. There also was no need for X-rays or specialists or a visit to "Disney Land". There was another unusual surprise, the blood could be drawn right then in her office. There was no need to travel to another carwash to get Gracie's blood drawn.

To treat Gracie's underactive thyroid gland, the doctor put her on Synthroid, a hormone replacement medication. There was no need to make a separate visit to a pharmacy. There was no need to take a sick child on yet another stop to get what she needed. And sit with her as you watch The Lucy Show. You know, watch a harried staff of pharmacists and assistants go through the Lucille Ball working on the candy assembly line routine as they try to fill one medication after another after another at an unbelievably hectic pace. No. The medication could be purchased at the doctor's office. And for six dollars for a month's supply.

There were no long lines leaving the doctor's office. Settling the modest bill was as easy as buying a cup of coffee as Starbucks. And it took just as little time and grief to schedule a follow up appointment for Gracie in one month.

The pleasant surprises from this medical encounter continued after we went home. The doctor *called us back* with the results of Gracie's blood test. It was the very next day. She told us it confirmed the diagnosis of hypothyroidism. There was no need for us to wonder for day after day what the blood tests would show. There was no need for us to call the office and fight with the phone queue to only leave a message for someone to call us back with the results. How incredibly user friendly and effective!

Then, a week after Gracie's visit, the doctor called us *on her own* to see how Gracie was feeling on her new medication and answer any and all further questions we had about her condition. She showed that she cared from start to finish.

I can imagine what you, the reader, are thinking. This was a one-time fluke. Or we have "an in," somehow, with Gracie's doctors. Or we belong to one of those super expensive upscale, monthly fee, medical practices. No on all three accounts. Sorry to play a trick on you, readers, so early in this book. But the real answer is that Gracie is our puppy and her doctor is the local veterinarian. That explains everything. I am sure those of you who have pets had have similar experiences when they become ill. I believe you would rate your experiences with your pet's healthcare providers as better ones than your own. The point I am trying to make is not that I am trivializing the importance of veterinarian medicine. It is just that I believe human medical care should be of the same ease, common sense, value, quality and sanity as for our animals. If veterinarian medicine works in this country, why not human medicine? If one system can function so well, why not the other similar one? Although we can learn a lot from how we take care of our pets to fix how care for humans is delivered, I am not proposing modeling American healthcare on the veterinarian medicine.

The medical care system in this country is broken. I am not sure we can even call it a system, the complex and loosely connected amalgamation of private and government insurers, huge health networks and solo practitioners and related pharmacological industries. That we do not even have an integrated plan, philosophy or system speaks volumes of how bad off we are. This book is about the problem and the solution.

I start by convincing you that our health system can do much, much better. I will show you although we as a country pay the most for our medical care, we get at best, middling results, and at times, Third World care, at worst. We then search together for possible solutions that would make all of us, healthier and live longer. Just as important, getting to that point must be less expensive and easier than it is today. It is my goal to open the debate about all aspects of American medicine. We will look, one by one, at the critical and yet unanswered questions about our healthcare system. Who should pay for it? How will we pay for it? What should be included in any healthcare plan? How can we be a healthier society? What incentives can there be to make us healthier than we are today? How can we improve the medical information highway? How can we reduce healthcare costs? How can we make the system simpler and easier to navigate? How can we change how healthcare is delivered to the patient?

I will pose each of these questions, look at all the possible answers and figure out which is the best one. My proposals are just common sense. But common sense often is what is most lacking in medical care. It reminds me of a tale from my childhood. When I would bring home a good school report card to my father, he would throw it back to me and say: "This is meaningless as there is no grade given in your school for common sense and that is what you need more than anything in life!" That may be my most important proposal for change in medicine. A dose of common sense. Let us do what makes most sense, based on the facts and alternatives that are available.

My lists of problems and solutions come from my 35 years practicing as a physician. As an introduction to you, I am a recently retired obstetrician-gynecologist. When I practiced, I felt there was a wall between my patients and myself. That the mechanisms that were meant to connect us and facilitate the delivery of medical care were in reality a Berlin Wall that had to be scaled. These first positive turned negative mechanisms included everything from medical insurance companies, to liability insurance, to hospital bureaucracies, to pharmaceutic companies to electronic medical records. I often pondered on how it should be better. I liked to brainstorm with co-workers and patients about it. I gleamed a lot from my experiences of 61 years being a patient or the loved one of a patient. Patients often forget that all doctors, at times, are patients. For I have been on both sides of the stethoscope and too many times knew I was part of a truly broken system.

Some of my ideas are radical. Sometimes it is better to start over again with something entirely new rather than tinker together a patch. We must not be afraid to try new things. Obviously, our present way of delivering healthcare is not working. Too much is at stake just to "keep on, keeping on" with what we are doing now. I believe that the right to be as healthy as possible is a fundamental right of all people. After all, is it not part of our heritage for all Americans to have the "right to life?" I hope, after reading this book, you will realize that American healthcare can be much better and demand fundamental changes.

1. IS AMERICAN HEALTHCARE BROKEN?

Let us start with the most fundamental question of all about American medical care. The first question we must ask is if there is a problem, at all. Is healthcare, as it delivered in the United States, as good or the best as it could be? You may say in any large endeavor, of course, there are things that could be improved. You might argue that things just need a little "tweaking." You may claim that we already have the best health system in the world. After all, we have the finest doctors, nurses and technology. Unfortunately, this is the response most Americans would give today. I answer back to you and them, if American healthcare is so wonderful, then why do we have the following problems?

For example, let us look at the local church where my family are members. For many years, the size of the congregation, the income from the donations from its members and expenses from running the church were steady. Suddenly over the past three years, the health insurance costs for the minister and tiny workforce have exploded. What was our church forced to do? The congregation had to dip into its emergency endowment fund, every year, to pay for its modest number of full-time employee's healthcare insurance. Think of the consequences for our small church. Money that is spent on health insurance is money not spent on missions to the poor, needed repairs to the church building, and for modest raises for the staff. In the long run, this pattern of spending for healthcare insurance is not sustainable and may be a reason why our church will have to close its doors.

If this were just a problem at our church, you may say "That's too bad" and forget about it and move on. But multiply the problem by the estimated 300,000 churches there are operating in the United States. If our church has this problem, they must face it, too. That is how many churches cannot completely fulfill their purpose because of the expenses of healthcare. Perhaps, you are not religious or even of a charitable bent. The problem is much bigger than that. According to the United States Small Business Administration, there are 28,800,000 small businesses (defined as having less than 500 employees) in this country. Each one of them faces the same medical insurance cost problem as our church. How do they pay for expensive, rapidly rising, and unpredictable cost of health insurance for their employees?

This problem then percolates in many directions through all parts of our country. It means fewer entrepreneurs wanting to start a business because of a huge initial fixed cost of health insurance. Maybe a future Steve Jobs or a Bill Gates will never get his or her start because of this obstacle. Established companies will hire fewer employees. Talented people looking for work are offered either part time positions or contract positions, because neither offer health insurance. The cost of the goods and services we buy are higher than they should be because these small businesses must pass on to us their high health insurance costs for their employees.

What is true for these small businesses is true for large ones, too. Having high health insurance costs for their workers puts them at a competitive disadvantage with similar companies in the rest of the world. As far back as 2004, the carmaker, General Motors, spent more on healthcare insurance for its workers than it did for the steel in its cars. How are we to compete with China and Germany in the business and industrial worlds, if our healthcare costs tie an arm behind our back?

For extremely high and unpredictable healthcare insurance costs, paid on behalf of workers by employers, makes American businesses and non-profit institutions much less productive than they should be. That effects every one of us, even if we never get sick one day in our lives. Healthcare in this country is not a system in isolation. For healthcare is intrinsically linked to all parts of the functioning of our society.

Here is a second example of a problem in American healthcare. As you have learned, I am a retired obstetrician/gynecologist. As every woman knows, an annual gynecologic exam is an important screening for maintaining her health. Because we can find and treat problems early, we can prevent serious medical problems later. This is the basis of preventative medicine. It is cost-effective, too, because the money spent on screening and early treatment is less than the money spent on treatment of advanced disease. It is better to fix a small leak in a roof than have repair the whole house. But almost every day that I practiced, I would witness that following surreal scenario. A woman would come in to the office for her annual checkup only to find that she was a day or two "early." That is because health insurances typically will pay for an annual exam every 365 days. Tough luck, if it is just 364 days. Just a minor inconvenience, you might answer? Think of the consequences of this seemingly *minor* inconvenience. The patient had to take at least part of a day off from work or arrange for childcare. She will lose even more time when she reschedules her appointment. The patient's appointment slot in the office schedule goes unfilled. That is one less patient who could have gotten care that day who needed it. The office staff must take time to reschedule an unhappy patient. Office staff are only human. The result of this and many such encounters per time makes them defensive, unpleasant and difficult to deal with. That is why a kind voice often is missing when you call your physician's office. That unpleasantness of the office staff means you are less likely to call the office when you need help.

You may say the solution to this problem is simple enough. The office staff should check when the patient was seen last for a checkup and schedule her appropriately, the first time. They try. Remember, though, not every insurance company has the 365-day requirement. For there are dozens of medical insurance companies. Plus, the same insurance company has different plans and these different plans have different rules. Patients change plans from one year to the next or if they change jobs. The rules of each plan change from year to year. It is impossible for receptionists, no matter how bright, no matter how well trained, to keep up with all these rules. And how can they expect our patients to know all the Byzantine rules of their health insurance? I was a physician and I never knew most of my own insurance company's rules.

And this is just one rule for one medical specialty. Medical insurance companies have hundreds of rules for each plan. Each insurance plan is always changing and different from all the others. Rules for which laboratory you can go to for bloodwork. Rules for how much your doctor's visit will cost you and how much they will pay the physician. For example, the same exact operation performed by the same physician will pay her a wide range of fees. Rules for which medical tests are covered by the plan and which are not. Rules for which medications are covered at which "tier," or level of preferred status. Rules for which hospital you must go to, if you become ill. Just don't become ill a thousand miles from it. I do not think I am telling you anything new, but it is funny that we as a society have accepted it. For it is like playing dozens of different games of Monopoly, each day, but with each game having a slightly different set of rules. Sometimes you collect $500 at Free Parking, sometimes, you do not. Except for this game, so much more is at stake that bragging rights to a boardgame.

Everyone in the American healthcare system, including the patient, must deal with a confusing and fluid system of private insurance rules. Let us expand this view of the rule labyrinth even wider. Almost half of the healthcare in this country is covered by a government plan: there is Medicare for the elderly, Medicaid for the poor, government employee plans, military veteran plans and active military plans. And yes, they have their own Monopoly game rules, too.

Let us think about that HIPPA privacy policy form that your physician's office hands out to you, each time you visit. Have you ever thought of the trees that have been killed just to create the paper used by all the medical facilities in this country to print just that form? I have. Let us assume it is just one sheet of paper per HIPPA form. We then multiply that by the number of physician visits in the United States per year. According to the Center for Disease Control, there were 884.7 million visits for 2014. Keeping our estimate on the conservative side, we are NOT counting non-physician visits, such as to the laboratory sites and hospitals that also give out these wasteful HIPPA papers. Next, we divide that figure by the number of pieces of paper that you get per tree. According to the nonprofit group, Conservatree, it is 8333.3. Pulling out your calculator, you will find that we kill 106,164 trees each year for those silly forms. Doing a little more math, if you factor in that there are 800 paper trees planted per acre (www.treeplantation.com), that is over 132 acres of trees.

Even a child would know an easy solution to this paper waste problem. If you want to require that one in a million patient who perhaps has been living on the dark side on the moon to know about his HIPPA privacy rights, you could simply require a sign be placed prominently in every office and medical facility. This is one tiny example of the next layer of the onion of complexity of American healthcare, the rules made by local, state and federal agencies that regulate it. Of course, it goes far beyond HIPPA. Medical care providers and patients are buried in paperwork. It is almost all redundant, wasteful, expensive and bad for the environment. Worst of all, it builds that wall. I call it the Berlin Wall of American healthcare. A Berlin Wall between the provider and patient that separates them which really should be a bridge. All the time and effort that should go to medical care instead is channeled into bureaucratic nonsense.

Let me give you a third example of what is fundamentally wrong with American healthcare. Do you know what one of the most dreaded questions you can ask a physician? "What are my test results?" It is not because we do not want to share them with you or explain what they mean to you. It is because we cannot find or at least easily assess them. For all the talk of the wonders of computerized medical records, it has not fulfilled its promises. Ask any physician and she will tell you it usually is more of a hindrance than a help. That is because there is no central depository for all your medical information. If I asked you for all your financial records, you could direct me to your Quicken or similar program, which has all your investments, banks, credit cards and loans stored to one place, even though they come from many different sources. No such program exists in this country for your medical information. Today, you, the patient, are on your own to compile a complete set of your very important health information.

Even within the same hospital, there are several separate databases or storage sites or programs. There may be separate ones for in-patient care, for the emergency room, for radiology studies, for billing and for physician offices. These programs must not like each other very much because they do not communicate with each other. It is obvious how this hinders your medical care. When a physician sees you, she does not have immediate access to all your medical information. She often must spend valuable time tracking down a critical piece of information, instead of taking care of you. The American Medical Association estimates that the average physician spends 52 hours a year just *logging on* all the various medical record systems. For it is far easier to get the local weather forecast in Nairobi than find the result of a blood test performed on a patient across the street from the office. Besides wasting time, this decentralized system leads to waste and more expensive medical care. For physicians, unaware that tests have already been performed, will order them again.

EMRs, as electronic medical records are called, are very difficult to use. This is because they must answer to many masters, none of whom are the patients. These include: medical insurance companies for billing purposes, governmental agencies that check on whether EMRs are being "used meaningfully" and the requirements of dozens of different medical specialties. They throw up too much distracting data at the healthcare provider. Using one is like driving through Times Square in New York City on a busy Saturday night. You cannot see where to drive because of all the flashing lights. Plus, they do not give you the important information that you need to know as if our car does not even have a speedometer.

Because of all the attention they require to use them, nothing in recent years has put more bricks in that Berlin Wall between physician and patient than the EMR. Today, having a conversation with your doctor is like trying to have one with a teenager with his nose buried in his iPhone. Both do not look at you, only at their glowing screen with a blank stare. You are not sure if you are being heard for you do not get even a nod of the head or the glance of an eye. The interaction has become much more impersonal, even sterile. Even more importantly, information is not being communicated. Remember almost all the information for making a diagnosis comes from the history, the directed story that the patient tells the doctor. If you and your physician are not communicating on some critical level, that information is not going to get to him.

The lack of any sort of integration between medical facilities extends beyond the medical records that demand too much attention and do not chat with each other. Let us say you have been having abdominal pain. You consult with your family physician. She orders some blood tests and an ultrasound test. Thinking you might have gallstones, she refers to you a general surgeon. Here is where the trip to Disney Land begins. At the family physician, at the laboratory drawing center that takes your blood, at the radiology faculty that does your ultrasound test, and at the general surgeon's office, you will have to repeat the same, bureaucratic steps over and over again. Negotiating with the phone tree to schedule an appointment, the insurance paperwork, taking time off from work, waiting for your appointment, waiting at the medical facility and explaining your problem over and over again. Like Disney Land, you must wait in a long, long serpentine line for the two minutes of what you came for. Then you must repeat it again for the next ride.

You may argue that I am a whiner. (I am, just ask my wife.) That I only see the glass half empty. That the American medical system has the best physicians and nurses in the world. That people come from all over the world for our cutting-edge care (Sorry for the pun.) That American pharmaceutical companies have developed most of the world's life-saving medications. That no other system in the world has the latest medical technology. That the American healthcare system, though not perfect, is like the German philosopher, Leibniz, said, is the "best of all possible worlds." That the faults that I have described are to be expected in any human endeavor. Okay, enough for the antidotes, let us look at the facts.

Let us judge American medicine in a way that medicine,

itself, judges whether a therapy is the best or not. Medicine judges if a medication, surgical procedure, or screening test is good based on whether it is "cost effective." Simply, it means, you get what you pay for. In cost effective terms, for $15, you would expect a mediocre steak, but you better be getting an incredible hamburger.

To find these statistics, you just go to WHO, the World Health Organization, which is an international non-profit with close ties to the United States. WHO gathers all types of health and medical care information from over 150 countries. Therefore, we can compare statistically American healthcare with the rest of the world and see how we are doing.

Let us start with the "cost" half of the "cost-effective" problem. How much do we spend on healthcare? To even out for different population sizes of different countries, let us look at how much is spent on healthcare per person for the year. Let us take the year, 2014, the last year there is data. What we discover is that the United States is number 1 of all of the countries in the world, at $9,403 per person. And it is way ahead of the rest of the pack. The number 2 country on healthcare spending per person per year is tiny Monaco at $7,302. Listed in table 1 are the top five countries and some other major ones.

Table 1. Spending (US Dollars) on Healthcare Per Person (2014)

Rank	Country	Spending
1	United States	$9,403
2	Monaco	$7,302
3	Luxembourg	$6,468
4	Switzerland	$6,468
5	Norway	$6,347
8	Germany	$5,182
11	Canada	$4,641
12	France	$4,508
14	Australia	$4,357
16	Singapore	$4,047

20	Japan	$3,727
23	United Kingdom	$3,377
190	Central African Republic	$25

You may argue, after looking at the data in table 1, that the United States is a wealthy country. It can afford to spend more on healthcare than the rest of the world. Then let us look at this data in a different way. Let us look at the percentage of each country's gross domestic product (GDP), or stated in another way, the percentage of the total value of all a country's goods and services, that is spent on healthcare. It is like looking at what percentage of a person's yearly income is spent on her car or his housing to determine if it is too much. Look at the statistics in table 2. Again, the United States is number 1. For the year, 2015, 16.9% of the gross domestic product went to healthcare, or more than one dollar out of six. Way, way behind at number 2 is Switzerland that spends 12.1% of its GDP on healthcare.

Table 2. Spending on Healthcare as Percentage of Gross Domestic Product (GDP)

Rank (2015)	Country	% of GDP
1	United States	16.9%
2	Switzerland	12.1%
3	Germany	11.2%
4	France	11.1%
5	Sweden	11.0%
6	Japan	10.9%
9	Canada	10.4%
12	Norway	10.0%
13	United Kingdom	9.9%
15	Australia	9.1%
-	Singapore	4.9%

It does not take an advanced degree in statistics to notice that by any measure that more is spent on healthcare per person in the United States than any other country. Therefore, at the minimum, we should have the best healthcare results, in comparison with the rest of the world. We should be the healthiest people on earth. We should not get hamburger results for the steak prices we pay.

Remember the money spent on American healthcare does not exist by itself in some big cookie jar, waiting to be used to pay our doctor bills. Money *spent* on healthcare is money our society *cannot* spend on other important things. Imagine for a moment that the United States spent as much money on healthcare each year as a percentage of its gross domestic product as the second country on this list, Switzerland. That somehow that if the Swiss could spend "only" 12.1% of their GDP on medical care, then we could limit our spending, too. It cannot be that farfetched. It is only a drop to the number two spender on our list. What could we do with the extra 4.8% of our GDP that we would save each year? According to the World Bank's statistics, the GDP for the United States in 2016 was $18.57 trillion. Therefore, there is a potential savings of 4.8 percent of that, or $891,000,000,000 ($891 billion). And that savings would accrue every year!

That is three times the total salaries and cost of benefits of all the teachers in the country. Speaking of education, we could send every student who wanted to go to college for free, nine times over! It is one-ninth of the amount of money required to properly maintain all our crumbling roads, bridges and infrastructure (Committee for Economic Development). Therefore, in nine years, we would be all caught up in maintaining our infrastructure. We could build 3,000,000 affordable housing units, every year! If you wanted to keep the money in a health-related field, we increase the amount of money the government spends on cancer research 90-fold. If you are of a frugal nature and do not want to spend the money, we could pay off the estimated $19 trillion of the nation debt in just over 21 years.

We could travel to Mars. We could rebuild our cities. We

could feed our poor. We could solve the problems of global warming and the rest of the environment. Let your imagination go wild for a minute. Just think of what you would do with those extra national resources. Economists, when they think this way, talk about opportunity cost. Money and resources saved on one thing is now available for another. Because we spend so much money on healthcare in the United States, it costs us in terms of all the things we cannot do. Remember, policies for healthcare do not live in isolation. What we decide to do and how we decide to do it for healthcare is intertwined with everything else we do as a society.

You may now say, "Sure we spend too much on healthcare, but we at least we have the best system in the world. We get what we pay for" Let us now turn our attention to the "effective" half of our cost-effective analysis. This is simple to do. There are dozens of parameters that measure how well a country delivers healthcare and we can compare them to our own. The easiest one to look at and the most basic healthcare statistic is life expectancy at birth. That is, how long, on average, someone who is born in that country, today, would expect to live. If a society provides for a good medical system, then that someone should live a long time. Table 3 comes from WHO and lists both the top countries and some other examples of countries lower on the list in terms of life expectancy for the year, 2015. It also compares it to how much that country spends on healthcare.

Table 3. Life Expectancy at Birth Versus Healthcare Spending as a Percentage of Gross Domestic Product in Selected Countries (2015)

Country	Life Expectancy at Birth Years, (Rank)	GDP % GDP (Rank)
Japan	83.7 (1)	10.9% (6)
Switzerland	83.4 (2)	12.1% (2)
Singapore	83.1 (3)	4.9% (124)

Spain	82.3 (4)	9.0% (40)
Australia	82.5 (5)	9.1% (15)
France	82.5 (9)	11.1% (4)
Sweden	82.5 (10)	11.0% (5)
Canada	82.2 (12)	10.4% (9)
Norway	81.8 (15)	10.0% (12)
United Kingdom	81.2 (20)	9.9% (13)
Germany	81.0 (24)	11.2% (3)
Costa Rica	79.6 (30)	
United States	79.3 (31)	16.9% (1)
Cuba	79.1 (32)	4.9%
Chad	50.2 (223)	

As you can see from this list, as expected, the richest nations populate the top of the list. The United States, however, is way, way down the list at number 31, between Costa Rica and Cuba, two just moderate-income nations. It is ironic when you think of it, that way. If we came in thirty-first in the Olympic gold medal count, this would be headline news in every newspaper (or its web homepage!) and there would demands for Congressional investigations. What this means, for all the money Americans spend on healthcare, we only get a so-so life expectancy out of it.

Let us drill down a bit and look at more specific measures of a nation's health. A commonly used one among investigators is infant mortality. This is the number of infant deaths that occur up to one year of age, per 1,000 live births. Listed in table 4 is such data, ranked by countries, from the WHO, for the year, 2015.

Table 4. WHO Infant Mortality Rankings for 2015
(Infant deaths up to 1 year old per 1,000 live births)

Rank (2015)	Country	Mortality Rate
1	Luxembourg	1.58
2	Singapore	1.77
3	Iceland	2.03
4	Japan	2.20

5	Finland	2.26
6	Italy	2.30
8	Norway	2.50
9	Sweden	2.80
14	Spain	3.00
16	Germany	3.10
20	France	3.34
24	Switzerland	3.68
27	Australia	3.96
29	United Kingdom	4.19
36	Canada	4.73
39	Cuba	5.50
40	United States	5.97
41	United Arab Emirates	6.23
174	Angola	96.22

Again, wealthy nations are the top of the list. And again, the United States is ranked below all the major rich countries of the world at number 40, just below Cuba. Remember there is more to this list than a bunch of numbers. There is meaning in human terms. Imagine for a moment an alternative universe where the United States' infant mortality rate is like that of Spain. Spain is not an extremely wealthy country. Their infant mortality rate of 3.00 deaths per 1,000 live births is just in the middle of the pack of developed nations at number 14. What that means is there would be 2.97 fewer infant deaths per 1,000 live births in the United States, every year. For 2015, there were 3,978,497 lives births in our country (National Center for Health Statistics). Doing the simple math means 11,816 fewer babies that would die, each year in the United States. Every year. That is between three and four times the number of people who died on the 9/11 attacks on our country. Every year, because of the inadequacies of our American healthcare system, we suffer the heartache of three to four 9/11 attacks, just in excessive infant mortality. Because these losses occur one by one and not in a large group, they do not draw the media attention of the losses of terrorism. But they are lives lost with all their potential of their lifetime and pain families in the same agonizing way.

Let look at another national healthcare statistic, for me a personal one, one close to my professional heart, maternal death rates. It measures how safe pregnancy and childbirth are in our country compared with the rest of the world. A little background history first. The huge decline in maternal death rates was one of the great victories of twentieth century medicine. In 1900, a mother had a one in a hundred chance of dying from a complication of pregnancy, labor or delivery. Today, in the United States, it is about one in 7,100. This is thanks to such advances as routine prenatal care, blood banks and antibiotics. But can we do better? How do we do as a country take care of our mothers in comparison with the rest of the world? Table 5 gives us this answer.

Table 5. Maternal Mortality Rates for 2015 (World Bank)
(Maternal deaths per 100,000 live births)

Rank	Country	Mortality Rate
1	Greece	3
2	Poland	3
3	Finland	3
4	Iceland	3
5	Belarus	4
6	Italy	4
11	Japan	5
12	Spain	5
15	Switzerland	5
18	Germany	6
20	Australia	6
25	Canada	7
29	France	8
47	Qatar	13
48	United States	14
49	Sierra Leone	1360

Again, this is a significant gap between the top, low maternal morality, rich Western countries and the only mediocre rate of the United States. Let us put this number into human terms. Think of how many mothers' lives we would save each year if we just could attain the relatively average for a Western country of Australia's maternal mortality rates. Doing the arithmetic of saving 8 lives per 100,000 live births, that would mean 318 fewer mothers would die from their pregnancies in the United States each year. That is more lives lost than die in our country from terrorism or school shootings each year. These lives lost are just a tragic as those lost from terrorism or school shootings. For they are sudden and unexpected, cutting short lives of mothers with families in the prime years of their lives.

Are you convinced yet we have a problem with American healthcare? Let us turn to see how our country does with behavioral and mental health. The WHO keeps data on the number of psychiatrists there are in a country per 100,000 people as a rough measure of the quality of mental health. Table 6 is from 2011, the most recent year they had data from which they had data.

Table 6. Number of Psychiatrists (2011)
(Per 100,000 population)

Rank	Country	Number
1	Switzerland	41.42
2	Monaco	36.47
3	Norway	30.77
4	Finland	28.06
5	France	22.35
12	Germany	15.23
16	Australia	12.76
17	Canada	12.61
33	Italy	7.81
34	United States	7.79
35	Slovenia	7.06
180	Eritrea	0.00

This time, at least, the United States is ranked with Western European countries. But it still quite a way down the list. We have only a third to half as many psychiatrists per capita as Germany or Canada. With all the problems our country has related and associated with mental illness from opioid addiction to gun violence, we certainly need more behavioral health specialists than we have today.

Let us turn to preventative health data. As a measure of this effectiveness, let us look at the immunization rates for measles. The WHO recommends all infants receive their first dose of the vaccine by age one year. According to the Washington Post article of February 3, 2015, 113 countries have higher immunization rates than the United States. Not just Europe does better than us, but countries such as Libya, Iran, Bolivia, Vietnam and Kenya. Low immunization rates lead to measles outbreaks, which unfortunately, we have seen too often in the United States. We should be ashamed of ourselves as a nation that we cannot do something so simple to prevent something so serious.

Next on our report cards of health care, let us look at statistics that measures the quantity of general medical care in the United States as it compares with the rest of the world. Table 7 lists one such simple measure. It is the number of physician visits per person per year in selected countries. The premise of this data is that the more access you have to health professionals, the more opportunity you have to get healthy. The data comes from countries that are part of the OECD, the Organization for Economic and Cooperative Development. They are a group of the 35 richest, democratic and free-market countries.

Table 7. Number of Patient Visits to Physicians per Person per Year (OECD Countries for 2015)

Rank	Country	Physician Visits
1	South Korea	16.0
2	Japan	12.7
3	Hungary	11.8
4	Slovak Republic	11.4
5	Czech Republic	11.1

6	Germany	10.0
11	Canada	7.7
12	Spain	7.6
13	Australia	7.4
	Average of All OECD Countries	6.9
16	Italy	6.8
20	France	6.3
29	United States	4.0
35	Columbia	1.9

In contrast to what we see when we visit our country's crowded physician waiting rooms, Americans just do not go to the doctor as much as most of the rest of the rich world. We see our physicians for almost 3 visits less per year than the average for the entire OECD. Why so few visits, even though our waiting rooms are full of patients? The reason for this discrepancy is simple. We do not have enough practicing physicians in the United States. This is demonstrated in table 8, which lists the number of practicing doctors per capita for countries in the OCED.

Table 8. Number of Practicing Physicians per 1,000 People (OECD Countries for 2013)

Rank	Country	# Physician/ 1,000 People
1	Austria	4.99
2	Norway	4.31
3	Sweden	4.13
4	Germany	4.04
5	Switzerland	4.04
6	Italy	3.90
7	Spain	3.81
12	Australia	3.39
17	France	3.09
21	United Kingdom	2.77
24	United States	2.56
28	South Korea	2.16

Table 8 shows that the United States has a severe physician shortage, in spite being a rich, developed Western country. Not having enough physicians means less care can be delivered. Less care for patients means we all are less healthy and do not reach our maximum health potential. There are detrimental effects from this physician shortage even when we do get medical care. Those physicians that do practice are overworked, prone to burnout, forced to take risky shortcuts and perform carwash line type medicine. Starting to sound familiar? No wonder we only get a couple of minutes with the Wizard of Oz.

There is a disjunct, here. We spend a lot of money on medicine, but we do not see doctors. If the money spent on healthcare in the United States is not going to patient visits, then where is it going? Let us look at the data for the number of CT scans performed per capita in those same OECD countries per year. This is compiled in table 9.

Table 9. Number of CT Scans Performed per 1,000 People per Year (OECD Countries for 2013)

Rank	Country	Rate
1	United States	240
2	Luxembourg	202
3	France	193
4	Greece	181
5	Belgium	179
13	Canada	132
	OECD Average	120
15	Australia	110
16	Spain	96
19	Switzerland	90
20	United Kingdom	76
23	Germany	62
27	Finland	32

If you live in the United States, you are twice as likely to have a CT scan performed on you as compared with someone in the rest of the rich world. This is despite the fact you are going to the physician less often. What does that mean? First, it implies patients in the United States, when they do go to their doctors, are sicker, and much more likely to need expensive technology. Which in turn means, they are getting less preventive care to avoid needing the advanced technology.

Second, at some level, this data means there are too many CT scans and other expensive tests and technologies performed in the United States. If the rest of the world is healthier than we are as measured by our many different criteria but, at the same time, the rest of the world uses less technology, that means we must be doing something wrong in American medicine. We are. We are substituting expensive and risky testing and technology for basic hands on physician care.

Why do substitute tech for touch? There are several intertwined reasons. The United States is unique among the medical care systems in the world in that it has a severe medical liability (malpractice) problem. So much so, there is a culture of fear among medical practitioners. If you could listen anytime to two American physicians discuss the management of a case, almost invariably the subject of malpractice is raised. Fear of a lawsuit enters every medical decision made in this country. No one performs well with a gun pointed toward their head. The tendency, therefore, is to do everything in a particular case. Order every possible test. Do the most advanced therapy, even if it is not the best one. It leads to the perception among health professionals that every patient is a possible future legal opponent. Obviously, that is not good for the rapport that is needed for the proper level of communication to get the right diagnosis.

Second, American physicians practice out of fear of failure rather than doing the truly right thing. That is why we do too many Cesarean sections compared with the rest of the world. We are loathed to try new techniques or think outside the box as we find medicolegal safety in conformity. We order too many tests, including CT scans, with the philosophy of "just to be sure" in a field of human endeavor where we can never be certain. We practice trying to create the persona to our patients that we are doing everything and anything all the time, rather than just doing the right thing.

Third, expensive technology becomes a shortcut solution for overworked, understaffed physicians. If Detroit wants to stretch the number of workers they have to build their cars, they add time-saving robots to the automobile assembly line. American physicians, burdened with time constraints, also turn to advanced technology as a substitute for one on one time with a patient. CT scans, MRI scans, blood tests and specialty consults replace the time it takes to get a good history.

There is a problem with these expensive tests, besides that they are well…expensive. These tests have risks for the patient. For example, using our CT scan example, the x-rays from the test expose patients to significant amounts of radiation. There is a significant rate of allergic reactions to the dyes used in the test. The biggest problem of all from such diagnostic test is called the "incidental finding."

Say you have a history of having kidney stones. You have suffered with them on many occasions throughout your life. You wake up one day with that severe flank pain, blood in your urine and nausea that you know is another kidney stone that you are passing. In pain, you make a trip to your local emergency room where they have treated you before. The emergency physician sees you and immediately orders a CT scan of your abdomen "just to be sure" you do have a kidney stone. (Because all of the moaning and screaming as you come into the hospital isn't convincing enough.) Sure enough, the CT scan shows that you do have kidney stones but wait. There is more. There is an "incidental finding" of a spot on your kidney. The emergency room physician treats your kidney stone and asks you to follow up with your regular physician about this kidney spot. Afterward, you feel better, but you have begun on your trip to Disney Land. First, the long line of scheduling an appointment, taking time off from work, waiting for your appointment and waiting at the office car wash to see your physician. When we see the Wizard of Oz, he says it is probably nothing but orders an ultrasound study of your kidney "just to be sure." (Oh, those dreaded words again.) Another line at Disney Land to schedule this test. More phone calls, more medical insurance hassles, more time off from work, all the time worrying that you are dying of cancer as you wait and wait to get the test. Finally, after you get the test, nothing happens. The silences from the system and the passage of time makes you certain that you are dying. Finally, after playing multiple rounds of phone tag with the office, your physician contacts you. That spot they found on CT scan so long ago is just a benign kidney cyst that you probably had your whole life. Sound familiar?

Studies show that 43%, almost half, of patients have an incidental finding when they have a CT scan of the abdomen. (This data is from: Frequency of incidental findings on computed tomography of trauma patients. West L Emerg Med 2010 Feb; 11(1): 24-2) Which means almost half of unnecessary CT scans start an expensive, stressful and potentially dangerous chain of further testing without making us any healthier. What is true for the CT scan is true for almost any medical technology testing.

Are you finally convinced we have major problems in American medicine? I hope you are not too surprised. Nothing in this chapter is new. I do not claim to be the prophet, only just another messenger of the crisis. Many other people and organizations have reached the same conclusions about the American healthcare system and its cost-effectiveness that I have. For example, there is the yearly Bloomberg Health Efficiency Index. It does a sophisticated analysis and summary of just how well fifty-five countries provide healthcare. It measures health bang for the medical buck. Getting used to seeing the United States at the bottom of the healthcare list? For 2014, we ranked 50th out of 55, between Serbia and Jordan. Part of that Bloomberg list is reproduced on table 10.

Table 10. Bloomberg Health Efficiency Index Rankings for 55 Selected Countries (2014)

Rank	Country
1	Hong Kong
2	Singapore
3	Spain
4	South Korea
5	Japan
6	Italy
10	Australia
14	Switzerland
15	France
16	Canada
19	China
21	United Kingdom
49	Serbia
50	United States
51	Jordan
55	Russia

The purpose of this first chapter is to convince you that we have huge and fundamental problems in the American healthcare delivery system. Reduced to the simplest form, we pay way too much for healthcare, the highest in the world, and we do not get close in services to what we pay. Continuing our earlier analogy, we pay surf and turf prices for day old leftover McDonald hamburger care.

(1.) Compared with the rest of the world, we pay more than any other country for healthcare, whether we look at the statistics on a per capita basis or a percentage of our gross domestic product.

(2.) If we measure healthcare effectiveness by how healthy a country we are, our statistics look like a developing to middle of the economic road country rather than a rich one. That includes such measures as life expectancy at birth, infant mortality and maternal mortality. There are many other measures of health where we lag rich countries in health, not mentioned in this chapter.

(3.) We lack basic, critical medical resources like number of physicians, mental health specialists and doctor visits.

(4.) We especially do a poor job when it comes to preventative health, as shown by our vaccination rates.

(5.) We have an overworked, burned out, logistically burdened, time pressured staff of physicians.

(6.) There is a cloud of medical liability that casts a shadow over every aspect of American healthcare. It builds a Berlin Wall between physician and patient, increases medical costs, and leads to unnecessary and often times, dangerous tests and procedures.

(7.) We substitute expensive technology for hands on care. This high-tech medicine does not always improve health. In fact, it generates a lot of further testing for chasing down "incidental findings." This leads to even more medical costs, risks and anxiety for us, patients.

Now that I have convinced you that we have a problem, let us logically explore how to fix our medical care system, step by step.

2. WHO SHOULD PAY?

We now agree there is a crisis with the American healthcare system today. Our first question in fixing it is a basic one. Who should pay for it? Today, when we hear discussion about who is going to pay, it is usually framed as a discussion about Obamacare. This is meant to be either a slur or a compliment to its chief proponent, the former president. The real name for Obamacare is the Patient Protection and Affordable Care Act. This was a law, signed by President Obama on March 23, 2010 that was an attempt to get more Americans either government or private health insurance. It tried to address the problem that so many Americans do not have insurance coverage when they become ill. It since has become a politically charged term, a dividing issue between Democrats who are for the plan and Republicans who are against it.

Let us reframe this debate. Let us get to the most basics of who should pay for healthcare in the United States. Let us discuss all the possible options and finally reach a conclusion of what we think is the best answer. For as a society, we must pay for whatever goods we consume or services we get. As my father-in-law, Bob Clark, always said: "There is no such thing as a free lunch." So really the question is when we talk about paying for something as a country, whether it be healthcare or anything else, is what pocket we are going to take the money out of.

Let us start with a simple, non-medical example. Pretend we need a new bridge. Any bridge provides a service, making it easier and less expensive for people and goods to move from one place to another. What would be the easiest and fairest way to pay for our bridge? Obviously, the bridge benefits its users, those that cross it. But even non-users of the bridge benefit from it. Items non-users buy cross it on the way to them. A new bridge may ease the traffic around where they live.

If you think about it, there are three possible answers to pay for our bridge. First, there could be a toll enforced on just the drivers who cross the bridge that covers the cost of the construction and maintenance of it. You might argue only those who directly use the bridge should pay for it. That this toll is fair to all of us. But is it the fairest or the best way? Remember, non-users of the bridge get benefits, too, by reduced traffic congestion and having their goods cross it. Plus, tolls are not an efficient way to collect money. It requires a lot of time and expense to collect it. You need to build a toll booth and hire toll collectors. There probably will be long lines to collect that toll, negating some of the benefit of having the bridge.

That brings us the second solution of paying for the bridge, a specialized tax. All those who choose to drive a car or other vehicle would be taxed to pay for the bridge, whether they used the bridge or not. This is the basis of taxes we have on gasoline purchases and driver and car license fees. You pay into a large pool of money that goes to all of the road and bridge construction and maintenance, whether you use a certain bridge or not. Since all drivers use some roads and bridges, it bundles the total cost and then distributes it among all the users. Is this specialized tax system on drivers and vehicles the fairest and most efficient? Probably not. For even if you do not own a car or ever drive, you still benefit from our new bridge and all roads and bridges. As mentioned above, the goods you use and other services that are provided to you came to you over that bridge or one like it. Plus, it is easier and less expensive for a government to collect a single tax rather than dozens or hundreds on all the shared resources we use.

That brings us to third solution to pay for our bridge. There would a general tax that would pay for all the common shared services we use as a society.

Notice, however we pay for it, our bridge is not free. Different people pay different amounts with each of the three scenarios. No solution can be completely fair to everyone. It is impossible to measure exactly how much each of us benefits from that bridge and charge us that exact amount for it. For example, the benefit that that bridge will vary over time. If you move away from the area of the bridge, you will derive less benefit. Rather than worrying too much about creating a funding of the bridge that is exactly proportional to those who benefit from it, it is a better use of our time to see what solutions are most effective in collecting the funds for the bridge. I hope you see that it is much more efficient (meaning less expensive!) to have one tax to pay for all shared services than a variety of specialized gasoline and car taxes or worse, go through the trouble of putting up toll booths and hiring toll collectors.

How does this bridge analogy pertain to funding healthcare in the United States? Like paying for the bridge, we can pay for our healthcare in one of three ways. First, we can pay for it like a toll. Every time you are sick or need a checkup, you pay for it out of your pocket. In medicine, this is called "fee for service." It is how most things and services are paid for in this country. It is like paying for a meal at a restaurant, a room at a hotel, or a new iPhone. If you want or need something, you pay for it directly. For most of the history, this is how we paid for medical services. On first glance, it seems like the fairest way to pay for medical care. Those who benefit from it, pay for it.

But there is an obvious problem with paying the toll for healthcare. Unlike a hundred years ago, modern medicine is very expensive. A single, unexpected illness can cost hundreds of thousands of dollars. Plus, healthcare is not an optional thing, like buying an iPhone (in spite the fact many of us say we cannot live without our smart phones). Insurance developed in the modern age as a way of spreading the high cost among potential users. That is why we have fire insurance, car insurance, homeowner's insurance and life insurance. We pay a small fee for these insurances every so often. Most of the time, we don't need the expensive service. But when we do, the large cost is paid by the insurance company that collects the fee or premium from lots of people. Smart math geek types, called actuaries, figure out the premium based on statistics on how often that the bad event might happen, whether it be a heart attack, car accident, house fire or early death. This is the second way of paying for the bridge. Just like paying a tax every time a driver buys gasoline, a fund is created for when a road needs repair or a new bridge needs to be built, funds for potential medical care are collected by health insurance companies.

Health insurance is so common and so talked about, today, you might think it always existed. But in the United States, it is a rather new concept, less than a century old. Blue Cross plans first started in 1929. They were medical insurance for hospital care. A year later, Blue Shield plans did the same thing for physician care. These were individual plans, meaning they were paid by the individual, just like most people pay today for car insurance. Eventually Blue Cross and Blue Shield merged into one big organization that granted franchises that covered different parts of the country. At first, Blue Cross and Blue Shield franchises were strictly non-profit agencies but as we shall see, that changed. Their goal was truly altruistic. To help people pay huge medical bills should the situation arise. The altruistic goal of the time is reflected by the fact that the Boy Scouts went around signing up members for their insurances.

Medical insurance did not become popular in the United States until World War II. And not for an obvious reason. During the war, there were price controls placed by the federal government on workers' wages to help prevent inflation that is so common during wartimes. To attract workers and pay them more without actually increasing their salaries, companies gave their employees, health insurance. It covered their and their families' medical expenses as a perk. This started the concept of group health insurance plans. They are called group plans because the company is paying the premium for a whole group of workers. Today, this is the most common way Americans get health insurance. In 2016, about 155 million, or almost half of us, get our health insurance this way.

After the war, people realized there was money to be made selling health insurance, both of the group and individual types. This led to the founding of the large for-profit health insurance companies we are familiar with today. These for-profit companies competed with the Blues. In fact, in 1994 Blue Cross and Blue Shield even allowed its franchises to be for-profit companies if they wanted.

There are a lot of advantages to this gasoline tax way of paying for the bridge or having employers pay for group health insurance for their workers. First, being a group plan, the rates are less expensive than for an individual plan. Most things, including insurance, are "cheaper by the dozen." Second, the health insurance plans, having lots of covered members, can negotiate with the different healthcare providers, including hospitals, drug manufacturers and physicians for less expensive rates for the services they provide. As large users of services, they can demand a lower rate. Again, things are cheaper by the dozen. Third, by having the employer pay for the insurance, it feels "free" to the employee. But this is just a warm and fuzzy feeling, with no basis in reality. Know that really, we are paying for the healthcare insurance with our toil. Fourth, the money that goes to pay for healthcare insurance is paid with pre-tax dollars. That means we did not have to pay taxes on the money first before buying it. That is unlike an iPhone that you buy with post-tax dollars. That smart phone might cost $1,000 but you perhaps had to earn $1,500 in wages first, paid taxes on those wages and have $1,000 remaining afterward to pay for the phone. You usually do not have to pay taxes on the money earned to pay for health insurance. But the biggest advantage of all is that you *do* have health insurance. Meaning, you have a means to pay for health expenses which can be unexpected, unplanned and huge.

Then what is wrong with our American system of employer sponsored health insurance to pay for our medical care? First, health insurance adds an unnecessary complexity to how healthcare is provided. There are so many ways health insurance can work, it is overwhelming for both healthcare givers and healthcare receivers. Alert. Alert, dear reader, it is going to get boring and complex for the next few paragraphs and please feel free to skip it or skim it. First, there are six basic types of health insurance plans: Health Maintenance Organizations (HMO), Preferred Provider Organizations (PPO), Exclusive Provider Organizations (EPO), Point of Service (POS), Health Saving Accounts (HSA) and Indemnity Plans (sorry, no three-letter abbreviation for this last one). A look at the history of medical insurance in the United States would show that some of these types of coverage have had their moment in the sun, only to be replaced by other forms.

An HMO is a plan where you only can see certain physicians and use certain hospitals and facilities that belong to the HMO. Your care is managed or controlled by a "gatekeeper," typically your primary care physician. She decides whether or not you get any further care beyond seeing her. For example, if you hurt your shoulder, you need your family doctor's permission before seeing an orthopedic surgeon. This permission slip is called a "referral." HMOs, like Beanie Babies and the Macarena, were mostly a 1990s thing. Because they were both so restrictive in giving out referrals and so poorly run, they went from being very popular to almost disappearing during this decade.

A PPO is a plan where you have more health coverage with a certain group of hospitals and physicians because the insurance company has negotiated a lesser rate with them. Hence, the terms "Preferred Provider." They still will cover you if you choose to go out of the network, but you will have to pay more when you do

An EPO is organized like a PPO except you cannot go out of your network for your medical care and expect any level of insurance coverage. Hence the "Exclusive" term is used in place of the "Preferred."

A POS plan is a hybrid between an HMO and a PPO. It works like an HMO when you go to a facility within the network plan and works like a PPO when you go out of the network. PPOs, EPOs and POSs are all the rage, today. With the coming of the millennium, they replaced the unpopular HMO plans.

An HSA is a low cost, high deductible plan where money is put aside for medical care for when you need it. When you get sick, you tap into that account.

Finally, there is an Indemnity Plan. This was the first type of medical insurance and is becoming a dodo bird in rarity, today. With an indemnity plan, there are no restrictions on where you go for healthcare and the insurance just pays part or all the care when you are sick, regardless of where you go.

Besides *types* of plans, there are four different *levels* of plans. This means different plans, offered by the same insurance company will cover a different percentage of your total medical care bills. Obamacare terminology gives the level of plans metallic sounding names. With a bronze plan, you will pay about 40% out of your pocket (or wallet) for healthcare, the silver plan

30%, the gold plan 20% and the top of the line, platinum plan, 10%.

Speaking of paying, even with the best platinum health insurance plans, you must pay some of your healthcare costs from your own wallet. There are four different fees you have to pay: premiums, deductibles, co-pays and co-insurance. With healthcare costs so high today, almost all employers require their employees pay part of the premium, or recurring fees, for their health insurance. These premiums are deducted from your paycheck, every time you get paid. Alternatively, if you are individual buying health insurance on your own, naturally you are going to pay for all of the premiums

Second, you must pay a deductible. For the first healthcare services you need in a given year, you pay, yourself and until you reach this dollar level. It is just like a deductible for car insurance. If your car is in an auto accident and there is $4,000 worth of damage, if your car insurance has a $1,000 deductible, you pay $1,000 and the car insurance pays the remaining $3,000.

Third, there are co-pays. These are fixed costs for routine care that you are responsible for. Even worse, they do not even count toward you meeting your deductible. A typical co-pay would be a $30 fee you would pay to see your family doctor when you get the flu.

Finally, there are co-insurances. These are a percentage of your healthcare expenses you have to pay for a medical service after you meet your deductible. Healthcare insurances do give you one break when it comes to medical expenses you must pay. There is a yearly maximum out of pocket amount that you can pay each year.

Why are there so many different ways for you to pay for your share of your health care, that is the part not covered by your health insurance? It is the same reason it is hard to figure out how much you are really paying for your cell phone or what all those fees are on its monthly service plan. It is the same reason your internet and cable service plans are so complex. It is the same reason the base price for a new car is meaningless. By chopping up the cost of an expensive item or service into smaller and confusing parts, it is trying to appear less expensive. Like a $20,000 car feels like it only cost the $20,000 base price though we actually paid $25,000 for it after options, strange dealer fees and complex financing. As medical costs skyrocketed in this country, the added expense had to be paid somehow. The medical insurance companies could not absorb the added costs and stay in business. The employers could not afford to pay more for the health insurance and stay in business. Guess who had to pay? The cost was passed on to us, the employees, in these various disguised ways.

See how complicated it is? But, wait, it gets worse. Remember, there are dozens of health insurance companies. Each has different types of plans, such as HMO and PPO, and each type of plan may have different levels of coverage. The plans differ, too, based on the employer, so just changing jobs brings another level of complexity for us. The plans usually change from year to year, requiring us to keep up with our plan. The plans all have different rules for what hoops you must jump through to get more than routine care. There are literally thousands of rule books for payment of medical expenses at any given time in this country. The plans require us, the insured, to navigate through the rulebook for our plan and we have to travel that path when we are least able to it. After all, we only use medical insurance when we or our family members are sick!

All these different insurance rule books create a massive amount of medical bureaucracy. Let me tell you a simple tale that I am sure will sound familiar to you. One day, I received a bill in the mail for a doctor's visit I had six months ago. I looked at the amount due and it claimed I owed $63.47. Knowing these bills are notoriously inaccurate, I checked it on line against the statement of my medical insurance company to see how much they claim I owe my doctor. They said $43.47. Anyone who knows me knows I am going to do everything in my power to pay the lesser amount. So, I called the doctor's office, negotiated the phone tree to their insurance person, and naturally no one answered my call. I left a voice mail message. Days later I receive a return call from that billing person at the office. Of course, the biller was rude, curt and condescending. And after 15 minutes of back and forth, we agreed to disagree. Like Don Quixote, I carried on my fight against the medical windmill. I called my medical insurance company. After negotiating their phone tree, waiting on hold, and giving them every piece of personal information about me, including my blood type (O negative) to prove that I was who I say I was, I was able to talk to someone about my bill. After a ten-minute discussion and explanation of my problem, the representative agreed that I only owed $43.47 and they would take care of it with my doctor's office. Hooray!

But wait. Remember that awful joke about the five great lies? One of them must be: "I am from a medical insurance company and I will take care your billing problem." A month later, I received a second bill from my doctor for the same services. And yes, it still claimed that I owed $63.47. Back to calling my medical insurance company. Back to their phone tree and FBI interrogation to get to talk to someone. Back to telling their representative my longer tale of woe. This time, the representative, after reviewing my case thought I only owed $20.00! Again, she claimed she will settle the matter with my doctor's office. But remember the five great lies! A few days later, the same rude billing person from my doctor's office called me. A hint, it is never a good thing when a medical billing person calls *you*. Of course, she had the same crass attitude as the first encounter. And again, we agreed to disagree about my bill after another 15-minute debate that made our last presidential debates seem like a love in. Finally, she decided to "cut me a break" and only charge me $43.47. I took the offer, figuring I would never get her down to just $20.00. End of story.

I wish this was a rare instance of such medical billing confusion, but I am sure you all have similar tales. It is more than a frustrating problem of life in the twenty-first century. Think of the time spent involving just twenty dollars that included myself, the billing department at my doctor's office and with the representative of the insurance company. Think of the money spent by the insurance company and the doctor's office arguing over $20. All because we have an overly complex medical billing and payment structure in the United States. I think of this medical insurance complex as a three-person chess game played among the provider of medical services, the medical insurance company and the patient. All three parties have a difficult game to play. For it takes a lot of time, effort and money to process our country's medical bills. Let us review this chess game.

It often starts before any medical services even are provided. The providers of medical services, first, must figure out if the insurance company will pay for their services. Because if they will not, they are not going to do the service, figuring they are not going to get paid. Nobody works for nothing. This process is what medical insurance companies call "pre-authorizations." This is their promise to pay for the medical service and it must be obtained before certain medical services are performed (Hence, the "pre.") For medical providers, pre-authorizations are not easy to obtain. They are dealing with a half dozen or more insurance companies and scores of medical coverage plans, all with different and changing pre-authorization rules. Pre-authorizations may take several phone calls, involve the transfer of medical records and dealing with differing levels of the medical insurance hierarchy. For example, a D and C, one of the most common operations in gynecology, took the pre-authorization personnel from my old practice about 45 minutes to 1 hour of time to go through the medical insurance hoops. That is more time than the operation, itself, takes, which is usually only 15 minutes!

Collecting payments is even more burdensome. The provider must collect from two parties: the insurance company and the patient. After the service is performed, the medical provider must issue a claim, which is just a bill to the insurance company to pay for the patient's service. As expected, the medical insurance company does not pay easily. Claims are the other half of the bizzarro medical billing world for medical providers. Claims, unfortunately, are not like your bill from your plumber. According to a 2011 Governmental Accountability Office study, up to 25% of claims, or these request for payments, are denied. There are many reasons for the denial, but commonly it is just a transcription error, a slightly wrong number entered into the computer system. That means phone calls and more computer work by the medical provider who is trying to get paid.

Medical providers also must collect fees from patients. Because of the complexity of co-pays, co-insurance and deductibles, few patients understand their medical insurance or have any idea in advance how much a medical procedure will cost. Most patients assume there will be no charge or a minimal fee. Multiple angry phone calls are made, daily, by patients to the provider because of the unexpected high costs. Medical bills have a high rate of being unpaid. Providers have to spend a lot of time and money collecting usually tiny amounts of money from a large number of patients.

The second player of our chess game, the medical insurance company, needs a huge labor force for both ends of the payment process. Thousands of employees are needed to enforce their own complex rules of pre-authorization and processing claims submitted by the medical providers.

The patient, of course, has it worst of all in this complex three-way chess game. The last thing they want to do when they or a loved one is sick is figuring out the complexities of their health insurance policy. If they are very ill, they are going to be bombarded with multiple bills. Being sick means also the loss of income and the often the inability to pay the bills. Bills go unpaid.

Imagine you suddenly develop a kidney stone, hundreds of miles from home. I have. Believe me, you would rather be in Philadelphia, my home town. Before you go for care, you realize, you must call your primary care physician to get permission to be seen in the emergency room. Then you realize that your care is not going to be covered very well since you were stupid enough to get sick far away from an in-network hospital as required by your insurance company. Then afterward, you get multiple bills from the different providers that took care of you: the hospital emergency room, the emergency care physician and the radiologist who read your CT scan to diagnosis your kidney stone. You are going to have to pay these bills. Back and forth you go between the different medical provider's offices and your medical insurance company's 800 number. One refers you back to the other. Every time you call, you get a different explanation. As you try to sort out all of these unexpected and complex medical bills, you are placed in collections. Then you cannot get a loan for a new car when you apply for one, months down the road, because this affected your credit rating. You are frustrated by all the time you lost dealing with what should be a simple matter.

The complexity of the three-way chess game opens the system for mistakes. According to Huff Post, at least of 30 to 40 percent of all medical bills have errors. And the Medical Billing Advocates of America say the mistake rate might be as high as 80 to 90 percent. The average overcharge by a hospital is about 26 percent according to M-Scribe Billing. These errors add up to unnecessary higher medical costs for the entire system. This is both for the overcharge errors themselves and the time for everyone in the chess game to fix them, if and when they are discovered.

You may argue, that we live in a complex, modern world. That you have the same problems dealing with bills from your cable and internet provider. (I know I do.) But this complexity of the American health care insurance system has a much higher cost to society. That leads us to the second problem with a private insurance model of healthcare payment. It is expensive. Very expensive. A big chunk of what you pay for private medical insurance goes to pay for the huge bureaucracy the medical industry created for itself. Let us look where a typical dollar of your healthcare insurance policy goes. This data comes from a report by the America's Health Insurance Plans, an association of private insurers, from March 2017. Only 79.7 cents of that dollar go to pay for the actual medical care. Insurers call this number the "medical loss ratio." Cynically, it demonstrates how (not) eager they are to pay for your health bills. About 2.7 cents go as a profit for the insurance company. Surprisingly, medical insurance companies are not cash cows like Google or Apple. The rest of that dollar, 17.8 cents goes to "operating costs," what it costs to run the medical insurance companies.

You may say, of course, it is expensive to run a private medical insurance company. They must pay thousands of employees to process claims, staff call centers and buy sophisticated computer systems. They also spend a lot of money on advertising and executive salaries, too. But can they be more efficient? Let us compare the operating costs of private healthcare insurance to a "has to be very inefficient" governmental one, namely Medicare. Bernie Sanders, when he ran for president in 2016, claimed it is just two percent. Silly, socialist Bernie. That number cannot be right. Yes, Bernie, the real number is only 1.4%. Medicare spends just 1.4 cents out of that one medical dollar to run its system versus 17.8 cents for private health insurance. This data comes from the 2017 Annual Report of the Boards of Trustees of the Federal Hospital Insurance and Federal Supplementary Medical Insurance Trust Fund. They should know the correct answer for they are Medicare's financial overseers.

Imagine the savings for the entire American healthcare system if insurance companies could be as efficient as Medicare, supposedly an "inefficient governmental system." Steffie Woolhandler and David U. Himmelsteind did. Their article of the April 18, 2017 in the Annuals of Internal Medicine, called "Single-Payer Reform: The only way to fulfill the president's pledge of more coverage, better benefits, and lower cost" estimated $504 billion each year. Think of what that huge number means. If it costs $9,403 to provide healthcare to one American, we, as a society, could afford to pay for healthcare for an additional 54,000,000 people, one-sixth of the population of the country.

Still, we are not finished with describing the unnecessary healthcare system costs from our inefficient "gasoline tax" model of payment. We have only dealt with the cost to the insurance companies. It costs a fortune for healthcare providers to collect the money owed to them from the healthcare insurers. Then they pass on those costs to all of us. There is a famous statistic, quoted by David Cutler, one of the world's leading healthcare economists from Harvard. He cites that the prestigious Duke University Hospital in North Carolina has 900 hospital beds but 1,300 billing clerks!

How much does it cost for the healthcare provider part of medical billing? An article published in 2014 estimates $248 billion each year with $70 billion spent in physician offices, $74 billion in hospitals and $94 billion in other health services (Jiwani, A, Himmelstein D., Woolhandler, S., Kahn, J. G. Billing and insurance-related administrative costs in United States' health care: synthesis of micro-costing evidence. BMC Health

Serv Res 2014: 14: 556.) The article estimates that 80% of these costs are wasted. That if we had a simple, single one-payer system, we could save $198 billion annually on medical billing.

This waste in administrative costs is confirmed by a study from the Harvard T.H. Chan School of Public Health, the Harvard Global Health Institute and the London School of Economics. They found such costs eats up 8% of our total health expenses each year, while it is only between 1% and 3% for our peer countries of Western Europe, Japan, Australia and Canada.

It is easy to bash American medical health insurance companies. Remember the Jack Nicholson movie from 1997, "As Good as It Gets" and how there were cheers in the movie theater when the characters took a swipe at HMOs? But they are only the iceberg of the medical administrative expense problem in the United States. For beneath the surface of the medical insurance companies, there often is another bureaucratic layer. The Economist (March 15, 2018 article) calls this hidden layer, the medical aggregators and includes such entities as pharmacy benefit managers and preferred provider organizations. You can think of them as hired subcontractors of the medical insurance companies. Although seldom seen and rarely discussed, these account for 46 of the America's top 200 largest health companies and account for 46% of all profits in the industry. Each American pay $200 a year just in extra profits that go to these shadowy middlemen. Are you starting to understand why the setup of the American healthcare is so expensive and not producing the results that it should?

So far, we have seen that a "gas tax," private medical insurance model of paying for American healthcare that we have today is complicated and expensive. A third and most serious problem with this model is that is does not cover everyone. Traditionally, to have medical insurance, you had to work for company that provided it to you or be a family member of someone who did. In 1965, Medicare was created as a governmental health insurance plan for those over 65. In 1972, the disabled and those on kidney dialysis were added to the Medicare program. Included in that same law that established Medicare, was Medicaid, health insurance coverage for the very poor. In 1997, the Children's Health Insurance Program or CHIP for short was started to cover children who did not have health coverage. These government programs, however, only filled some of the gaps in our country's medical insurance coverage. It still left millions of people without insurance. They may be the unemployed, those who work for themselves, work part time or work for small companies that do not give their employees health insurance. Many are "contract" workers, who do not receive health benefits. Those without insurance typically "took their chances" as individual health insurance policies were too expensive.

Obamacare's main purpose was to give more of these uninsured people group medical insurance. Under the plan, more people qualified for Medicaid. Those without insurance who were not eligible for Medicaid could buy it online at insurance "exchanges." These are federal and state governmental websites that brought together individuals buying insurance and private medical insurance companies offering different plans. To encourage people to buy medical insurance, it became a law that most people had to have it or otherwise they paid a fine. This part of Obamacare is called the individual mandate. Also, people with a lower income received a lower insurance premium, with the rest subsidized by the government. Obamacare did succeed in its primary goal of getting more people health insurance. In 2010, before the act came into effect, 48 million Americans did not have coverage. In 2016, that number dropped to 28.6 million, according the New York Times article of May 22, 2017.

Then why isn't everyone singing Obamacare's praises? After all, so many more people are insured. Three reasons. The program, like gun control and abortion rights, has become a symbol of the divide between the left and the right in our country. In all such lightning rod cases, emotions have replaced compromise and common sense. Second, Obamacare keeps intact the messy, complex, expensive private healthcare insurance system. It did nothing to address spiraling healthcare costs and has contributed to its out of control cost spiral. And third, there still are many, many people in the United States without health insurance.

You might be a little mean and ask why should we care if "other people" do not have health insurance? "After all, you are insured." Remember, we all are just a change of life situation away from losing this critical protection. Divorce, loss of our employment, disability and changes in the political situation in Washington can happen. No one is secure.

Unpaid healthcare bills are the number one cause of bankruptcy in the United States. This is according to a 2013 study from NerdWallet Health, which analyzed data from the United States Census, the Center for Disease Control, the federal court system and the Commonwealth Fund private foundation. About 2 million bankruptcies each year are due to unpaid health bills, ahead of those caused by credit card debt and home foreclosure. In addition, 15 million other people will deplete all their savings trying to cover their medical bills. Another 10 million will not be able to afford their rent, food and utilities because of them. Even having medical insurance does not protect against these financial calamities. This is the problem of being "underinsured." Many people's health insurance coverage is so porous, they still accumulate huge health costs in the forms of copays and coinsurance.

A more selfish reason you should care about the uninsured and underinsured is that those who do pay their medical bills ultimately pay for those who do not. The loss from uncollected medical bills naturally is passed on in the form of higher medical rates. It is just like the honest customers ultimately pay for the items stolen by the shoplifters. And it gets worse. The uninsured forego preventative care. This includes such services as mammography, blood pressure screening and eye examinations. Also because of the high associated costs, they do not have close monitoring of their chronic diseases, such as diabetes and asthma. This is a penny wise but pound-foolish approach because they are more likely than the insured to show up with more advanced stages and therefore have more costly forms of disease. They are less likely to have a consistent set of medical providers. This leads to inefficient evaluations and treatments and duplication of testing. The uninsured are more likely to use expensive emergency services. They wait until they get extremely sick and then must to go somewhere. Since emergency facilities, by law, must treat them. There is where they go. By trying to save money, they spend more healthcare dollars which are passed on to the insured. This is not an attempt on my part to "blame the victim" but rather blame the system that creates such awful dilemmas in healthcare choices for so many Americans.

There is an inherent unfairness in how the uninsured are billed. Medical care providers, whether they be a physician's office or a hospital, have a fee schedule for the cost of the services they provide. When you first look at one, you are shocked by how expensive these fees are. That is because they are the retail prices. Like the sticker price of a new car, few people pay at these rates. That is because the medical providers have a negotiated price with the medical insurance companies. The providers must accept this wholesale price, regardless of what they bill from their fee schedule if they "participate" in the health insurance plan. And almost all American physicians participate in several plans. That means providers are paid at many different rates for the exact same service. The fee schedule retail price may be up to ten times what the providers accept from the medical insurance plan. However, the uninsured do not have that luxury and are stuck with the full retail price.

The biggest reason we, who are lucky to have medical insurance, should care about those without it that they are less healthy than us. Steffie Woolhandler and David U. Himmelstein found such in their September 19, 2017 article in the Annuals of Internal Medicine, "The relationship of health insurance and mortality: Is lack of insurance deadly?" People with health insurance have 0.71 to 0.97 relative risk of mortality compared with those without. These numbers mean that everything else being equal, the uninsured have a 3% to 29% increased chance of dying compared to the insured. This simple statistic goes a long way in explaining the contradiction between Americans spending more on healthcare than anywhere else in the world but receiving only so-so health services. The uninsured are underserved and we have a lot of people who are uninsured.

Having a large group of less healthy Americans affect all of us. Sick people are less productive. They miss work and cannot readily perform the routine activities of life. They make us a less efficient society. Cars do not get built. Meals are not cooked. Computer programs do not get written. There are delays in filling orders. There is a need to pay someone else for overtime. We all pay indirectly when one among us is sick. Again, I am not trying to blame the victim, just stating the fact that our medical care system is unfair to all of us. For having so many people uninsured deprives us of the future services of a potential movie star, professional athlete, judge or physician, all of whom could have enriched our society in a thousand different ways.

This speaks of the callousness and shallowness of our modern American society. By not insuring everyone in it, we are saying we are willing to throw away millions of years of lives to be lived. That we are willing to accept unnecessary pain, suffering and heartbreak. That we can be blind to preventable human suffering and premature death. I think we are a better people than that. Some things are fundamental human rights: free speech, freedom of worship and access to clean water and adequate nutrition. It is about time we add the right to healthcare to that list. If the Founding Fathers of the United States were alive today, I think they would agree with me.

That leads to the third and last way that a society can pay for that bridge. It can collect one general tax from everyone. Since we all either directly or indirectly derive benefits from the bridge and it is impossible to measure how much that exact benefit is for each of us, we each should pay for it and pay for it according to our means. By simply collecting a simple tax in the most efficient matter, in the long run we save money on funding for our bridge. I see you reading between the lines of my last statement. Yes, I am making a case for universal health coverage.

What does universal health coverage mean? Americans have a confused picture about what that term means. We, too often, reflectively think of it as something evil. Let me describe the elements of this model and see if I can change your mind. If we look at countries around the world, we see there are four basic models of paying for and delivering healthcare. The first is the out of pocket model. It is the toll at the bridge model described above. It is where people do not have any health insurance and pay as they go when they get sick. It is what is seen in poor regions of South America, Africa, India and China. It was what was seen in this country before the 1920s and 1930s. And it is what is seen for the uninsured in United States to this day.

The second model is the Bismarck model. It is the named after the Prussian chancellor who united Germany in the nineteenth century. He was the first world leader to start a system of health insurance, financed by the employer and employee jointly. The differences between this system and the private insurance system we have in the United States is that the "sickness funds," as the insurance entities are called, provide universal coverage and they do not make a profit. The Bismarck model still is found in Germany and also found in France,

Belgium, the Netherlands, Switzerland, Japan and Latin America. Note with this system, like that of the United States, the actual medical care is provided by private hospitals and physicians.

But the Bismarck model is a huge step forward in creating a significantly healthier society compared with our country in that its medical coverage is universal. It still has the disadvantage of complexity with multiple insurers and high bureaucratic costs. Bismarck model countries have healthy populations, ranking among the top countries in health outcome statistics. However, they have high healthcare costs even though they rank behind (way behind) the United States. This is shown with the data in table 11. It gives two statistics for four Bismarck model countries: their rank among countries of the world in health spending per person and their rank in life expectancy.

Table 11. Spending and Life Expectancy for Selected Bismarck Model Countries

Country	Rank in World for Health Spending Per Capita	Rank in World in Life Expectancy
Switzerland	2	2
Germany	3	24
France	4	9
Japan	6	1
AVERAGE	3.75	9.00

The third model of a national healthcare system is the Beveridge model. It is named after William Beveridge of England who created the British National Health Service. Here, the government provides as well as pays for the healthcare of all its citizens. The government collects taxes and creates and runs health facilities to provide it. Most physicians and other health care providers work for the government. As a side note, there usually is a small, "private," cash-only parallel system, too. It is for those, usually wealthy patients, who do not want to deal with the governmental one. The Beveridge model is what most Americans think of when they think of "socialized medicine" or national health insurance. Today, the Beveridge model is found in Great Britain, Spain, Scandinavia, New Zealand and Hong Kong. Believe it or not, we have small scale Beveridge systems in the United States, today. There is the Veterans Health Care Network, where retired military personnel have access to their own separate healthcare system which they do not have to directly pay. Also, there is the active military health care system and the Indian Health Care system. The model creates low costs and a healthy population. You can see this by looking at the data from selected Beveridge model countries table 12.

Table 12. Spending and Life Expectancy for Selected Beveridge Model Countries

Country	Rank in World for Health Spending Per Capita	Rank in World in Life Expectancy
Great Britain	13	20
Spain	30	4
Norway	21	15
New Zealand	24	17
AVERAGE	22.00	12.00

With Beveridge plans, like the Bismarck plan, there is universal coverage. Healthcare is considered a right and no one goes without it. People who live under a Beveridge system like it. For example, The British like it so much they bragged about their system during the opening ceremonies of the 2012 Olympic Games in London.

The system does have its problems, which is why I am not advocating for it. Access is the biggest one because the government controls the supply of healthcare. For the government decides how many physicians to hire, how many clinics there are, and what other facilities are available. Also, to control costs, facilities are drab and crowded. Now you know why the American Veterans Health System is always in the news and gets skewered for the care it gives.

The last model is a true National Health Insurance model. With this model, there is just one national insurance, funded by taxes and run by the government. However, the actual medical care is given by independent providers and private hospitals. There is universal coverage. Everyone in the country has medical insurance. This last model is seen today in Canada, Australia, Taiwan and South Korea. If you think about it, American Medicare is a National Health Insurance model. National Health Insurance results in outstanding health for the population, because everyone has coverage. It has costs that are lower than the Bismarck model because having just one insurance makes the whole system more efficient. Patients and healthcare providers only deal with one entity. Also, the governmental insurance has tremendous leverage over costs. They are the only game in town buying health services, so they can negotiate from strength to keep costs down. That is why so many Americans cross the border to Canada, just to get their medications, many of which were created in the United States. Its efficiency and effectiveness is demonstrated in table 13 which shows the costs and health outcome for selected National Health Insurance countries.

Table 13. Spending and Life Expectancy for Selected National Insurance Model Countries

Country	Rank in World for Health Spending Per Capita	Rank in World in Life Expectancy
Canada	11	12
Australia	14	5

South Korea	19	11
AVERAGE	14.67	9.33

Access usually is not a problem in countries with a National Health Insurance because there is a free market component on the supply side. If there is a demand for more physicians and hospitals, more providers can enter the market to provide for such services. It is no different than if the demand for hamburgers goes up, more McDonalds will be built. For proof of this, you just have to go back a chapter and remember South Korea, a country with such a model of health care, has the highest per capita number of physician visits per year in the world!

My conclusion for who should pay for healthcare is to fairly tax everyone to pay for the bridge since we all directly or indirectly will benefit from it. But let the builder and maintainer of the bridge be the private sector. The data bears this out. Table 14 shows the average spending and life expectancy of the different national healthcare models. With the National Insurance Model, you get the results of the Bismarck Model for less cost.

Table 14. Spending and Life Expectancy for Different National Healthcare Models

Model	Average Rank in World for Health Spending Per Capita	Average Rank in World for Life Expectancy
Bismarck	3.75	9.00
Beveridge	22.00	14.00
National Insurance	14.67	9.33

I hope my logic has shown you that the solution of who should be for the American healthcare system is a single payer, universal, National Health Insurance model. Let us review the reason why this is the best solution. First, one payer simplifies the system for everyone, whether you are the patient or the provider. It is simple because there is just one set of rules everyone follows.

Next, this model will cost less than what we have now because it eliminates the private health insurance middleman and the shadowy medical aggregators, and the costs associated with such as a system. Plus, the governmental single payer will have tremendous leverage in what it pays to the providers. Finally, it saves money in the long run by providing more preventative services and earlier therapies.

Because of the universal coverage aspect of the model, we will be a healthier country. This is not only good for those of us who now do not have insurance and suffer the ill health consequences. It also is good for the rest of us, because we gain their productivity that is lost today because of preventative sicknesses. Under such plan, we will be a more productive and happier society because of the effects of this "trickle down health."

On the surface, our day to day medical care would look similar to what we have now. You still would see your independently employed physician and have care in your private, local hospital.

We, when we are patients, will be happier with the plan, too. In fact, there was an accidental experiment that proves how happy we will be with it. In the United States, today, as we have seen, we are an unintended laboratory for healthcare care systems as there are examples of all four possible models. In 2015, the Gallop Organization did a poll on how satisfied Americans were with their present health plan. The answer depended upon which of the four models they had. Not surprisingly, the uninsured were the least happy with a satisfaction rate of 41%. If the respondent had an individual health care plan that they paid for themselves, the happiness rate rose to 65%. That number went up further to 69% if they were covered by their employer's group medical insurance plan. But guess who among us was most satisfied? Those with their medical coverage by the government were the happiest of all. The satisfaction rates for Americans with Medicaid, Medicare, and active or retired military coverage were 75%, 77% and 78%, respectively. The irony is that all four groups are seeing the same medical providers and having care at the same hospitals.

Finally, and most important of us, I am convinced that the providing universal medical insurance is morally right thing to do.

Let me hear your objections. I see all those hands of yours going up out there. *Number one.* My taxes will go up and we can never afford this a plan. That is partially true. Taxes will go up to pay for it. But, as we shall see in the next chapter, not as much as you would think. But most importantly, in the long run, the plan will save you money. Right now, we pay more as a country for healthcare than any other by any judgment criteria. But we pay for it in a confusing piecemeal way like we pay for our cell phones and their service plans, that hides the true total cost. For we pay through reduced wages because our employer provides for some of our healthcare insurance. We pay through further reduced wages for the rest of our healthcare insurance that is deducted from every paycheck. We pay out of pocket costs for coinsurance, copays and deductibles. We pay federal taxes that pay for Medicare and Medicaid for the health insurance for the elderly and the poor. We also pay through our federal taxes for the health insurance for the active and the retired military. We pay through our federal, state and local taxes for private health insurance of the government employees at all three levels. Finally, we pay higher costs for all our goods and services to pay for the healthcare insurance of the workers that supply them to us. Because a National Health Insurance plan will take a smaller bite out of our gross domestic product, we all will be richer.

Number two. You say that it is not fair to the healthy to have to pay for the care of the sick. As we saw with our bridge analogy, it is impossible to quantify how much of a common service, an individual uses. Therefore, no system of healthcare payment can be completely fair on a pure monetary basis. But remember everyone eventually gets sick and remember we all are just a heartbeat away from a life altering and very expensive medical illness. We all someday will use this coverage. For everyone paying into a common pool to help those who might need it, including ourselves, is the basis of any insurance, whether private or governmental.

Number three. You feel that the government should not be involved in healthcare. For it messes everything up that it touches. You have tattooed to your forearm, Henry David Thoreau's saying: "That government is best which governs least." Guess what? You are way, way too late. The government already is involved in healthcare and is in it, big time. A study in the American Journal of Public Health from 2016 calculated that the government already pays 64.3%, almost two-thirds, of all healthcare costs in the United States. It pays for Medicare, Medicaid and active military insurance and the Veterans Administration. It pays the health insurance premiums for public employees' private healthcare insurance. Through Obamacare, it subsides the private healthcare premiums of many more.

Already, the government pays more for healthcare as a percentage of the gross national product than any other country in the world, including all of those who have total governmental involvement! For the United States government is the biggest spender on healthcare on an absolute basis and a per capita basis than any other government of any other country in the world. Therefore, if our government is going to pay for healthcare, let it spend our money in a more efficient manner.

Number four. You feel that National Health Insurance is a

form of socialism. It creates a welfare state, and that is just not America. If by socialism, you mean the government taking care of certain basic services for all its citizens, we have been a welfare state from the beginning. Certain services run more efficiently and effectively by the government. If you think about it, that is why we have a government. These services include a military to protect us from foreigners who want to do us harm, a police force to protect us from the evil doers among us, an educational system to make us a more productive workforce, and a highway system so we can move around.

We already have a "socialized" healthcare system in the form of Medicare for the elderly and disabled. There is not a politician in Washington, no matter how right wing, that would advocate to dismantle this "socialized" system. So, you cannot use what I call the Communist "pink-o" argument.

Number five. You argue that the government is not good at running things. My response is that the government is not good at running *some* things. For there to be an effective American National Health Insurance, the federal government would have to do two major things, correctly. First, it would have to collect taxes to pay for it. Fortunately (or unfortunately, depending on your point of view), the government is very good at this task. According to an article in the Los Angeles Times from March 31, 2015 by Doyle McManus, the Internal Revenue Service, the main collector of federal taxes in our country, is the model of efficiency. It collects more taxes with less people each year and does a better job in comparison with similar tax agencies in the rest of the world.

The second thing the government would have to do if it had to run a National Health Insurance is properly administrate it. Luckily, it has had practice. It already is doing so with Medicare, and it has fifty plus years of experience under its belt. We have already seen that Medicare is already a model of efficiency in that is spends less than two cents on the dollar for its own costs, much more efficient than private health care insurers.

Number six. You worry that there will be long waits to see doctors and then you would not be able to see the doctor you want to see. Remember, I am not proposing the government take over the healthcare *provider* side of medicine. There still would be private hospitals and private practices. Only the provider of insurance would change. (I do not think too many people will miss Aetna, Humana or Blue Cross, too much.) There is no reason to believe hospitals would shutter their emergency room doors or doctors would start selling pencils on the street corner instead of what they do today. As we have seen in countries like South Korea that already have a National Health Insurance with privately employed providers, they have some of the highest number of doctor visits per capita in the world. Instead of the number of doctor visits going down, I believe they would increase, especially for today's uninsured. Plus, having a *national* health insurance would eliminate the restrictions so commonly seen in today's private health insurance plans where a patient is limited to certain hospitals and certain providers. There would be no more worries about that unplanned kidney stone, 500 miles from home!

Number seven. You feel that there will be bureaucratic "death squads" that would prevent you from getting the care that you need. Guess what? They already exist with private healthcare insurance plans. All private plans limit what kind of care they will pay for and therefore you will receive. Private insurance plans limit how often you receive preventive care. For example, a woman cannot have a routine gynecologic examination more often than yearly. Private insurance plans must approve coverage for anything beyond basic care. As we have seen, if you need your gallbladder removed, you need preauthorization by them, so they will pay for it, afterward. Private plans place medications in tiers, deciding to what extent they will pay for each drug. Private insurances limit coverage on experimental or non-mainstream procedures. To some extent, these measures taken by private health insurers are reasonable to keep healthcare costs in check. However, today's system is open to abuse. There are horror stories of patients denied coverage for very necessary care.

Having the government in charge of what will be covered has two huge advantages over the present system. First, there is uniformity. Every citizen has identical coverage. That eases the bureaucratic burden on everyone. There is no playing our insurance game of three-way chess with hundreds of different sets of rules. Second, patients will have more leverage. Presently, there is not much a patient can do if they do not like the final decision of their private health insurer. With a potential governmental insurer, the insured are in sense the bosses of the system, too. The ballot box and the representatives we choose can change any unfair restrictions on getting medical care. Because the rules for coverage will be nationwide and universal, any unfair restrictions will be quickly discovered and therefore, quickly corrected.

The rest of this book will go into the details of my National Health Insurance system proposal. Since I will be referring to the plan so often, it needs a name. Like almost everything in medicine, it has a name based on an anacronym. I call it the SPUN Health Plan, short for Single Payer Universal National Health Plan.

In concluding this chapter, I hope my data and arguments have convinced you that a single governmental payer or insurer of healthcare with universal coverage and private providers is what this country needs to provide for the best healthcare results, a more efficient system and reduced total cost. In the next chapter, I will talk about how we will pay for it.

4. HOW WILL WE PAY?

In the last chapter, I proposed a plan I called the SPUN Healthcare Plan to fund for all healthcare services performed in the United States. It is a government-provided, single payer, universal plan. This chapter explores the most logical way to pay for such a plan. Our funding system should meet the following three criteria. First, it should be a simple system, to collect from who is paying for it. Obviously, that is something missing in today's complex, multiple medical insurances mixed with various government programs which involves multiple layers of taxes, payers, payments and fees. Second, it should be efficient in collection, meaning it should not cost a lot of money to obtain the funds. For today, we as a society pay too much out of our medical dollars just to shuffle around and pass on medical dollars to the insurance companies and government programs. Finally, it should be fair as possible to all of us, who are paying for it.

The obvious answer to pay for a governmental health insurance program is through taxes. Taxes are society's means of having everyone chip in for services we all use, whether it be that bridge we have already spent too much time talking about in the last chapter, a police department or a public-school system.

Of course, everyone hates taxes, and everyone especially hates taxes that they, themselves, must pay. But if we want these services that benefit all of us, we must remember the old saying. Taxes, like death, are a certainty of life.

Taxes can meet our criteria for a good payment system. They can be a simple system. They can be efficient in not costing a lot to collect them. Finally, taxes can be a fair way of paying for healthcare since we all pay taxes and we all use healthcare services. We must, however, pick the correct tax plan.

Let us next discuss what would be the best tax plan to pay for our SPUN Healthcare Plan. Meaning, what are the best taxes? The rules for good taxes are like the rules for a good medical payment system. The taxes for our plan should be simple, and efficient in collection, and fair in what each of us pays. I want to add a fourth important criteria. It should provide incentives for us to do good things and disincentives to discourage us from doing bad things for our health.

Simple taxes mean they are easy to understand. After all, one of our goals of remodeling American healthcare is to make it simpler. What would be the best way of taxing based on this criterium? I propose using existing taxes, the federal income and corporate tax system we already have. Why add to the complexity of our world by creating a new tax? In fact, it would be simpler than our present system since we could eliminate today's Medicare tax on wages because we would no longer need Medicare! The collection of taxes and total operation of the system will take place only at the federal level. Again, why get the states involved and set up an unnecessary system of 50 separate healthcare programs? One tax that we already have, one level of government to collect and administer it to fund one insurance across the country. Simple, right?

You may be surprised to hear that there is not a separate tax for our SPUN plan. We don't need a separate tax just for healthcare insurance. After all, we do not have a separate tax for our national defense or one for our national parks or one to fund the Supreme Court. All those needed funds come out of the same big pot. Our National Health Insurance would be just another item in our federal budget, varying year to year in how much it would cost, just like all the other items in the budget.

Because the Internal Revenue Service would be collecting the needed revenues for the SPUN Health Care Insurance, it would meet the second goal of the ideal tax for it, it would be efficient in the collection. Relative to other countries, the IRS is very good at what it does, collecting a substantial proportion of what is owed to the federal government in a very cost-effective manner. Of course, you can argue that our present federal tax code should be simpler, easier to understand, and it should be easier to file our taxes. I agree with you totally but that is a subject for an entirely different book!

Having our proposed National Health Insurance as part of the general federal budget, paid by personal and corporate taxes would be a fair system, too. Everyone who works or gets an income from other sources must pay federal taxes. As mentioned above, since everyone would be covered, it is fair that almost everyone would have to pay. There would be exceptions. Those who are disabled, retired, unemployed or do not have other significant income would not have to pay. That is because they do not have the means to pay. But they still would have health insurance. You may say that is not fair to the rest of us. But already do this in so many other areas. You still have police protection and you still can use the roads, even if you do not pay taxes. This would just be another extension of the basic principle that we, as a country, take care of the disadvantaged among us. Plus, remember, giving the poor insurance saves the system money in the long run, by making them healthier and not needing more expensive services for advanced diseases.

Our present day federal individual tax system is progressive. That means, not only do the wealthier pay more in taxes, they pay more as a percentage of their income. This, too, is the fairest way of paying for our proposed SPUN Healthcare Insurance. It has been a foundation of our tax system from the beginning that those of us lucky enough to be successful should contribute more back to society. Wealth would be the only determining factor in how much you pay for healthcare. No longer would older Americans, those who work for themselves, those in work for companies who provide slim coverage of group healthcare, those with pre-existing medical conditions pay more than the rest of us. Today, it is random what each of pays for our health insurance. When arbitrary groups of people pay more for health insurance, that is an unfair system and that is what we have today. This unfairness of what you pay for healthcare in the United States would disappear by having it funded by the general federal tax system.

Businesses would pay their fair share for the plan, too. Why? They benefit when their workers are healthy. Plus, businesses will be getting a huge break in my proposed system by not having to pay for medical insurance for their employees. They also will save huge human resource costs in the paperwork and bureaucracy they need today to run their group medical plans. Think of all those open enrollment forms, work health fairs and other "fun" activities that would be eliminated each year. Businesses, especially small and growing ones, will be more likely to hire new workers when they need them, not having to worry about the costs of the fringe benefits of healthcare insurance. There would be less need for part time workers and contract workers, schemes today's businesses have evolved to avoid medical insurance costs. Workers' unions around the country would have less reason to strike as they would not have to battle businesses over ever shrinking medical coverage.

A good tax code does more than collect taxes, simply, easily and fairly. It encourages people who pay it to do good things and avoid doing bad things. For example, there are tax laws such as for 401k plans and Individual Retirement Accounts that motivate us to save for our retirement. The tax laws reward us for donating to charitable causes. They reward home ownership as this is an American ideal. On the other hand, today's tax system discourages cigarette smoking by placing a high tax on tobacco products and consuming too much alcohol by the same method.

Our future tax code, after SPUN takes effect, should do the same thing for our health by encouraging healthy behaviors and discouraging bad health practices. There are some baby steps toward that goal that exist today. As mentioned above, there are substantial taxes on both tobacco products and alcoholic beverages. In some cities, like Philadelphia, there is a soda tax to discourage the consumption of sugary drinks. Such "sin" taxes would work best at the national level, since people could not just drive a few miles down the road to purchase not-taxed soda out of the area. Suggested future taxes include ones on junk food, fast food and even sugar, itself. On the other hand, there should be tax credits for healthy foods and activities that encourage exercise. For example, there could be a tax break for businesses that either have gyms on site or pay for gym memberships for their employees. Developers could get a tax break from the federal government for building hiking trails and constructing bike paths. Throughout the rest of this book, I will detail many other tax code incentives and disincentives.

I know that you are worried about how much the SPUN Healthcare Insurance will cost you. And how much your taxes will go up. Yes, to pay for the plan, you will have to pay more in taxes. But remember, we already are paying for healthcare, just from many other different pockets. Converting to a single payer system and single financed system will save you money in other ways, more than offsetting any rise in your taxes. First, you will get a raise since the company you work for will not have to pay for your group health insurance. Second, your part of your medical insurance costs will go to zero. Third, unlike today, the part of your medical expenses you pay after insurance will be minimal. Finally, the costs of all goods and services, not just medical ones, will be lower since business will not have to pay for health insurance for their employees and they can pass their savings on to the costumer.

I can prove it to you. Let us do "back of paper napkin," that is, rough calculations of the future costs of health care. Let us do these calculations two ways. First, let us look at how the proposed plan on a macroeconomic scale of how it would affect the federal budget. Then, let us look how the plan on a microeconomic view. That is, its effect on several, different, but typical Americans' budgets. To do these calculations, we start with a couple of simple but plausible assumptions. First, the federal government will be paying for all American healthcare costs. That is easy to assume because we devised our healthcare plan that way. Second, the plan would lower health spending, as a percentage of our gross domestic product, to the level of the present day, second place country, Switzerland. This is very reasonable and in fact is on the conservative side. Conservative? I see you raising your eyebrow in disbelief. First, our federal government likes to spend more money than it takes in. This is called deficit spending. Therefore, it is unlikely that if the SPUN plan was enacted, that the government would pay for all the medical spending at the time it was spent. Second, we are aiming for the health spending rate of Switzerland. Switzerland does not have a single payer governmental funded health insurance plan. It spends, relative to income, a lot of money on healthcare, compared to the rest of the world. We can do much better than Switzerland, if we were to try. Therefore, the potential savings probably is a lot more.

Let us start at the governmental level "back of the napkin" calculations. Today, we spend 16.9% of our gross domestic product on healthcare or roughly $3 trillion. (Yes, the "t" in trillion is correct.) If we reduced this spending to 12.1%, Switzerland's level of healthcare spending, that annual amount would be reduced to $2.1 trillion. That also is the amount the government would have to spend each year since it is paying for the entire healthcare tab. Now remember the United States government at all levels already pays for 64.3% of all healthcare costs through programs like Medicare, Medicaid, present and retired military, the Indian Health System, and Obamacare subsidies. That amount, today, (64.3% times $3 trillion) is $1.9 trillion. Therefore, the extra amount each year that the government would have to pay would be the difference of the anticipated spending of $2.1 trillion and the amount it pays today or $1.9 trillion. That number is "only" $0.2 trillion or $200 billion. That is the amount we would have to pay by an increase in taxes.

Yes, $200 billion is a lot of money, but as a percentage of the federal budget, it is not that much. For 2018, the federal budget will be about $4.1 trillion, so the increase in the federal budget would be only 4.8%. For example, compare that figure to the cost of the very wasteful wars in Afghanistan and Iraq that have costed $5 trillion since 2001 or $294 billion a year.

That means our taxes would only have to be increased 4.8%. Remember we are making the very conservative assumption that the government, as it should, would pay for all the National Health Insurance, as it came along, rather than adding it to the ballooning deficit. Keep that percentage number of 4.8% in your mind because that is the percentage we are going to assume our individual and corporate taxes will go up each year.

We now move from the macroeconomic to the microeconomic by examining the future healthcare finances of some typical Americans under our SPUN plan. Let us begin with my son, Matt. He is 25 years old, single (and available). He works as a trader for a large mutual fund company and earns about $60,000 a year. His medical insurance is covered mostly by his employer. Like most millennials in their 20s, he is lucky enough to be healthy and only occasionally goes to the doctor, just for check-ups and such. Right now, he pays $6,100 a year in federal taxes, $3,720 for Social Security taxes and $870 for Medicare taxes, for a total of $10,690. (Please note these are not really my son's real personal financial numbers, but I am using him as a typical example of a young, single adult *and* to get his name in my book.) Thus, under my SPUN plan, I would expect his taxes to go up 4.8%, which is an extra $513, for a grand total of $11,203.

How does that compare to the total cost of medical care and taxes that he is paying now? The average American who has a group employer health insurance plan pays 17% of the cost of that plan. The average cost of the health insurance for a single person covered under such plan is $6,251. Therefore, today, he pays $1,062 a year for his portion of his health insurance. Being young and healthy, his out of pocket costs are low, just $300 a year. Adding up his present taxes and healthcare cost, he now pays $12,052. That is $849 more than he would pay under my plan. I am assuming, too, that his employer does not pay him a dime more, even though they probably would since they would not have to pay for his medical insurance anymore. And I am not counting on the money he would save on paying less or goods and services from companies that would have lower costs, being free of the burden of employee medical insurance.

Millennials, such as my son Matt, need and deserve a break. They live at a marked disadvantage under today's financial rules and circumstances. As a generation, they are saddled with debt from college student loans which boxes them into a financial corner. Their entry wages are being eaten up with spiraling healthcare costs. They must pay for part or all their health insurance coverage. They pay significant taxes for the healthcare of others including for Medicare and Medicaid program. Since most of them are healthy, they do not use much of the health services for which they pay. The SPUN Plan gives their generation a needed financial break.

Table 15. Combined Healthcare and Tax Savings under SPUN Plan for Matt (Young, single, healthy adult working for large company, now with group health insurance.)

Plan	Today	Proposed
All federal taxes	$10,690	$11,203
Health insurance costs	$1,062	$0
Other health costs	$300	$0
TOTAL TAX AND HEALTH CARE COSTS	$12,052	$11,203

Next, let us move on to my niece, Karen and her family. Karen and her husband, Page, are forty-somethings with two grade school age children. Both work, but Karen carries the medical insurance for the family. She is one of the few lucky remaining Americans who pays nothing out of pocket for her family's health insurance as she is a public-school teacher with a strong union and a great contract. Together, they earn $120,000 and have the dream upper middle-class life. They do have the expected health expenses of a young family including pediatric care, allergy shots, minor orthopedic injuries, trips to the emergency room for stitches and routine checkups. Let us look at how their medical finances would change under our SPUN National Health Insurance Plan. Today, they pay $12,453 in federal taxes, $7,440 in Social Security taxes and $1,740 in Medicare taxes for a total federal tax bill of $21,633, each year. Their proposed taxes would go up 4.8%, or an extra $865 for a future total federal tax bill of $22,498.

They still come out ahead, financially, under the SPUN proposal, though they do not have to pay for even a small portion of their healthcare insurance. That is because a typical family of four now pays $1,214 a year in co-pays, co-insurances and deductibles. That gives them a total health and tax cost of $22,847, as things now stand. All those co-pays for allergy shots and trips to emergency room and medications quickly add up, even for a relatively healthy family with great medical insurance. Again, we not counting on the possible increase in Karen and Page's salary from their employers not having to pay for medical insurance and the savings from the lower cost of goods and services they purchase.

Union members and others in our society with excellent and no out of cost medical insurance do not want to rock the boat when it comes to changing the present healthcare set up. After all, they feel like they get their healthcare for free, already. And how can you beat free? However, even with great insurance coverage, their direct costs for medical care is high as those copays and coinsurances costs are significant, even for them. Also, they have high indirect costs for healthcare in the form of taxes for the governmental medical programs and the higher price of goods because of the cost of inefficient and expensive healthcare for the workers who produce their goods.

Table 16. Combined Healthcare and Tax Savings under SPUN Plan for Karen and Page (Upper middle income family of four in excellent health with excellent medical insurance.)

Plan	Today	Proposed
All federal taxes	$21,633	$22,498
Health insurance costs	$1,062	$0
Other health costs	$1,214	$0
TOTAL TAX AND HEALTH CARE COSTS	$22,847	$22,498

Our next analysis is of the medical finances of my personal physician, Dr. Hal. He is a family physician with a wife and two teenage children. His wife does not work outside of the home. Hal is employed by a small medical practice. Today, they partially pay for a very basic Silver Level health insurance plan. He earns $225,000 a year, which is the average for his specialty. Being a bit older than Karen and Page, Hal, his wife and family, although still healthy, require more health care services each year. Ah, the joys of aging! Playing the same game, we have been playing, they now pay $35,957 in federal taxes, $7,936 in Social Security taxes and $3,262 in Medicare taxes for a total federal tax bill of $47,155. Under my proposed plan, their taxes would go up 4.8% or $2,222 a year for a total of $49,277.

Ironically, and there is so much irony in the setup of our present healthcare system, even though he is a physician, he must pay a lot out of his pocket for his share of his employee health insurance. Also, his plan's coverage is mediocre. This is because most physicians work for small businesses. Small businesses cannot keep up as well as large corporations with the exploding cost of health insurance for their workers. They compensate by asking their employees to pay a lot more for health insurance each year and by lowering their coverage. The typical small business pays only 65% of the $16,625 that is costs to cover the health insurance for a family of four. That means Hal must pay $5,819 in health premiums, annually. Plus, he pays double in deductibles, co-pays and co-insurance costs compared with Karen's family or $2,428.

That combines for $8,247 in today's total direct medical costs or $55,402 with taxes. Therefore, even a very well-off family, who would have to pay the most in taxes under my plan, still come out ahead. The upper-class fear taxes. They view higher taxes as a threat to their life style. What they should fear even more is the spiraling costs of medical care as this is more of a threat to their way of life. After all, they are the small and large business owners that must deal with health insurance costs for their employees and themselves.

Table 17. Combined Healthcare and Tax Savings under SPUN Plan for Dr. Hal (Upper income family of four with basic health insurance, high out of pocket costs.)

Plan	Today	Proposed
All federal taxes	$47,155	$49,277
Health insurance costs	$5,819	$0
Other health costs	$2,428	$0
TOTAL TAX AND HEALTH CARE COSTS	$55,402	$49,227

Next, we move on to my brother-in-law, Steve. He is a single, self-employed contractor and builder. Being single, without dependents, he "takes his chances" and does not pay for healthcare insurance, as it is too expensive. He earns $50,000 a year. This is not a lot of money but under the present rules it is too much as a single person to qualify for a medical insurance rate reduction under Obamacare. Steve would rather pay the small penalty of $695 than $5,692, which the average cost that a single person must pay each year for the bare bones Bronze level of health insurance coverage. He pays an additional $5,639 in Federal taxes, $3,100 in Social Security taxes and $725 in Medicare taxes. That is a grand total of $9,464 for his total federal tax bill, not including the Obamacare penalty. Under the SPUN Plan, his taxes would go up $454 for a total of $9,918. That is less than what he pays today for the penalty. Even though he is healthy and foregoes as much healthcare as possible and when he does need care, he goes to low cost clinics. He still spends $1,500 a year on healthcare. In a "good (lucky?) year," that means he spends a total of $11,659 for taxes and healthcare. Of course, he realizes he is just an appendectomy, which can cost up to $200,000 without health insurance, from total financial ruin.

If upper-class businessmen feel the weight of growing healthcare costs, middle-class self-employed ones now are being crushed by it. They face the dilemma of either having no medical insurance and having an illness that would financially destroy them or pay high, unsubsidized rates for low coverage under Obamacare and not have ends meet.

Table 18. Combined Healthcare and Tax Savings under SPUN Plan for Steve (Single, self-employed contractor without health coverage in good health.)

Plan	Today	Proposed
All federal taxes	$10,159	$9,918
Health insurance costs	$1,062	$0
Other health costs	$1,500	$0
TOTAL TAX AND HEALTH CARE COSTS	$11,659	$9,918

My Aunt Gloria is a wonderful example of aging gracefully that we all aspire to. She is 92 years young, still drives, is intellectually engaging and even travels around the world. She has a sharp mind and wit to match it. Being over 65 years old means she is on Medicare. As anyone on the plan knows, having this plan does not mean her worries for healthcare costs are over. She spends the Medicare average of $3,045 per year on medical costs. This is much less than the tiny tax increase she would have to pay each year under my SPUN Health Insurance plan. (See table 19.)

Table 19. Combined Healthcare and Tax Savings under SPUN Plan for Aunt Gloria (Widowed person on Medicare in excellent health.)

Plan	Today	Proposed
All federal taxes	$6,500	$6,812
Health insurance costs	$0	$0
Other health costs	$3,045	$0
TOTAL TAX AND HEALTH CARE COSTS	$9,545	$6,812

Medicare has been a wonderful plan for the elderly and the disabled. It is so popular, politicians are loathed to tinker with it. It gives us a glimpse into what a government, single payer, private provider healthcare system would look like in our country. It proves that we could be happy with "socialized medicine." But it has its problems, big ones, as it stands, today. About one-quarter of all people on Medicare or 15 million, total, spend 20% or more of their income on health costs each year. That amount includes costs for Medigap insurance, which is private health insurance to fill the "gaps" that Medicare does not cover. Medicare has significant co-payments. It does not cover dental, hearing and vision care. Although prescription drugs were added to the plan in 2006, the elderly need to buy a separate private plan. In addition, Medicare is a complex plan for members to navigate. For example, participants must pick from a variety of confusing coverages, each year.

But the biggest worry my Aunt Gloria or any of the elderly face is how to pay for long term care, should they need it. This is not covered by Medicare. The present American healthcare system is not facing up to the crisis that is growing each day as 76 million of us baby boomers age. We all are at risk for the need for long term medical care as dementia and other chronic illnesses become more common as we get older. Approximately 47% of aged men and 58% of aged women eventually will need long term health care. The cost is astronomical, typically costing

$80,000 a year for a shared room at a typical skilled care facility. Medicare and private health insurance plans do not cover any of these costs. There is long term care by Medicaid for the poor. In fact, Medicaid is the default payer of long term care for 61% of all patients in such facilities.

Therefore, today, only the wealthy and the poor can afford long term care. The middle class has the option of special long-term health care insurance, but it is very expensive and seldom purchased. Most people in the United States who need long term care will have to wipe out their lifetime savings and place a fiscal burden on their children. Then when they are financially ruined, they will become wards of the state, having their care covered by Medicaid.

Any society can be judged on many parameters. One of the most important judgments is how we treat our elderly. Our lack of a compassionate plan for taking care of the neediest of the elderly, those in long term healthcare facilities, as things stand today, would give us a grade of an F. Any solution for our healthcare system must provide for long term care insurance. Therefore, it must be included under the SPUN Plan.

Let us change gears a bit and look at the effects that the SPUN Health Insurance plan would have on businesses. We already have seen how our present system hurts small business owners. Now let us look at the businesses, themselves. My first example is the firm that does my accounting. It is not one of the "Big Four." It is a tiny, local company with just 100 employees. It has approximately $15 million dollars in revenue for its services, each year. On the expense side, it pays $1,500 per month for each of its 75 full time employees for just a mediocre Silver Level family coverage. That works out to $1,350,000 in health insurance costs or 9% of its total revenue. Like most small businesses, it tries to keep its insurance costs low by using this bare bone plan, hiring part time employees and even using some contract employees for whom it does not have to pay any benefits. The partners, when deciding on whether to expand its workforce, are slow to hire new employees, fearing the burden of paying for their medical insurance. Even when it does, good workers are reluctant to join the company, given its mediocre health benefits. They continually must balance their prices for accounting services, keeping them high enough to cover the huge medical insurance overhead but low enough to compete with the big accounting firms.

Sure, SPUN Health Insurance might increase my accounting firm's corporate taxes. But on the other hand, it would be free of the yoke of providing health insurance for its workers. Let accounting firms do accounting. Keep them out of healthcare. Freed of such responsibilities. it could hire full time employees much more easily, which would be good for the company and good for the potential workers. It would make the accounting firm more competitive with the huge firms. Its customers, too, would benefit from lower accounting costs for its services.

Finally, let us take a look of an example of a huge corporation, the Ford Motor Company, the car manufacturer. It, of course, is the famous company founded by Henry Ford in 1903 and is responsible over the years for such iconic American cars as the Model T, Thunderbird and Mustang. It is the second biggest car manufacturer in the country, behind GM and the fifth largest in the world. The estimated health insurance costs for Ford's employees are easy to estimate. The average cost for health insurance per worker for a family plan for a large company was $17,983 per year in 2015, according to the Kaiser Foundation. Businesses paid $13,390 of that premium on average with the rest coming out the employee's pocket. Let us assume that is what Ford paid. It is probably more as car manufacturers pay more because of long-standing union contracts. Ford has about 100,000 employees in the United States. That means it spends about $1.3 billion on healthcare insurance each year. It sells 2.6 million vehicles in this country each year. That works out to $515 of employee healthcare expenses per car or truck sold. No wonder new cars cost so much.

Ford and other large companies use different strategies to try and reduce their employees' medical insurance costs. They are paying less and less of the premium of their employees. In addition, to paying more of the premiums, employees are expected to pay more of their actual health costs, in terms of deductibles, co-pays and co-insurance. Large companies have the option of moving their operations to other countries, where health insurance costs are much lower. In Ford's case, this means Canada, a country which already has a National Health Insurance.

Despite these measures, this means Ford is less competitive with foreign car manufacturers who do not have Ford's burden of huge employees' health insurance costs. Ford must charge more for its cars. Our present health care system means we all lose at the corporate level. Ford, the company, loses. Ford's workers lose. Ford's customers lose by paying more for their products.

Hopefully you can see from these sample calculations of the medical costs for different people and different businesses, virtually everyone "wins" with our proposed SPUN Health Insurance plan. Though there is a small increase in our taxes to pay for it, there is a huge net decrease in spending on healthcare. We all would have more money in our pockets. That just makes sense. If you spend less money on one thing, you have more for another. If you spend less money on rent each month, you have more money for vacations. You may say there is no free lunch, that my National Health Insurance cannot save society that much money and give good healthcare. The following chapters will detail the plan's coverage and its savings. Stay tuned.

4. WHAT IS COVERED AND HOW IS IT COVERED?

You may be wondering what your health insurance and medical care would look like under our proposed SPUN Health Insurance plan? Surprisingly, it would not be that different from your present employer provided private insurance. Not only would it retain the good parts of the present system but there would be enhancements, too. For example, if you wish, you could choose and change your private physician, hospital and other health care providers, just like you can today. As an enhancement, you would not be limited in which providers you choose. All insurance created networks and other systems of preferred providers would be eliminated. You would not have to fear that kidney stone far from home.

It would be a simple Indemnity Plan, meaning fee for service. SPUN would pay your healthcare providers for each service you needed. In this sense, it would be much like an old fashioned Blue Cross/ Blue Shield plan of the mid twentieth century. There would be no restrictions or other hoops you would have to jump through to see specialists. There would be no need for paper or electronic referrals or other whips that HMOs use today to control access. It simply would pay a fee for the services you used. Remember, simplicity is the goal of our plan. For a simple plan is easy for everyone involved to use. It is easy for everyone to understand how payments works. Perhaps, most important of all, a simple plan saves money for the entire system.

Continuing this theme of simplicity, everyone in the United States will have the same SPUN insurance plan with exactly the same benefits. With everyone operating by the same rules, it makes it easier to move the huge bureaucracy that is American healthcare providers. By everyone, I mean, everyone. It would be same plan for children and adults, the disabled and the retired. It would be the same for those who work and those who do not. It would be the same for the wealthy one percent, the poor and all of us in between. It would be the same insurance for active military and retired. This plan would eliminate the thousands of different health insurance plans, all with slightly different payments and different benefits. Think of how easy it would be under this SPUN plan to be a medical claims processer!

It would get the government out of providing healthcare for it would eliminate such systems as the military veteran's system or Indian Health Services. You might think my plan gets the government too involved in healthcare. Actually, it would remove it from having to provide services, allowing the private sector to be the only game in town.

The SPUN plan would have not net out of pocket costs for us. By that, I mean, the sum of the medical expenses for everyone would equal the sum of health payment rewards. Yes, rewards. It actually would pay you for certain good health things that you would do. More about these rewards in a little bit.

There would be only three kinds of out of pocket health expenses. The first would be for some rare, non-covered services, like for purely cosmetic surgery. Sorry, that Botox for your crow's feet would not be covered under SPUN. I will go into detail later in this chapter as to what services would be covered and what would not.

Our second set of out of pocket expenses would be reasonable co-pays. The purpose of these co-pays is not to generate a significant revenue stream for the medical care system. It is just to have each of us stop and think before we go to the doctor or seek out other healthcare. It is human nature to take more of something than what we need when it is *completely* free. On the other hand, it should not be so much that it impedes people from seeking medical care when they truly need it. This was the original purpose of co-pays when they were introduced by HMO health insurance plans, decades ago.

The amount of the co-pay that you would pay should go up with the intensity of the care that the patient is seeking. Under any medical insurance system, you do not want patients running off to the emergency room the first time they have a minor, tension headache. It should encourage us to see our primary care physicians as much as possible when we are sick. This makes sense since our family physicians, internists and pediatricians know us and our families best. And since most medical problems can be handled by them, it would be most efficient for the system to utilize their services as much as possible. Therefore, when we seek out care from a primary care doctor, our SPUN co-pay would be at the lowest price tier, a modest fee of $25.

Next up the ladder of intensity of medical service would be seeking out the services of a specialist. That copay would be $50. Again, it is higher, so we seek out our family physician, first for most problems. We should be encouraged to see our family doctor for our tension headaches, first, rather than running off to a neurologist. Notice this feature of the SPUN plan is not much different than what we are used to, today, with most group medical plans.

Have you noticed that urgent care medical centers have popped up suddenly all over the place? They remind me of when I was a child during the 1960s and hamburger chain restaurants, like McDonalds, seemingly appeared, like magic, on every corner overnight. Such care centers have flourished because they fulfil an unmet medical need in this country. Sometimes we have a minor medical emergency like an ankle sprain. But it is a weekend and our family doctor's office is closed. We know if we go to a regular emergency room, it is going to be both very expensive and it will be a much more time-consuming process than it need be. Urgent care centers fill in that middle ground. The co-pay for their services under our SPUN plan would be $100. This is lower than the proposed co-pay for a true emergency room, but higher than for a family physician or a seeing a specialist. Again, this is our system encouraging us to seek out the lowest intensity of care, as possible that the medical situation warrants.

Of course, there will be times in our lives when the services of a true emergency or trauma center are critical. The co-pay for such services would be $200. When you visit an emergency room today, you can see a vivid snapshot of what is wrong with our present-day healthcare system. Before you enter the building, you will see the sign for it advertising its services outside of the main hospital or medical center written as "ETC." This is short for Emergency Trauma Center. I think the ETC under today's American healthcare system has come to mean "etc.," short for the Latin word, "etcetera." The emergency room has become more than a place you go when you have a myocardial infarction or fall off the roof of a building. It is the place to go for medical care when there is no other place to go. It is like that junk drawer we all have in our kitchen that we toss in all the stuff for which we cannot find another logical place.

For example, the uninsured use the emergency room for simple and minor ailments or for neglected once minor ailments that are now much more serious. They go there because, by law, emergency rooms must take of everyone who presents to them, regardless of their ability to pay. Please do not take this as an example of me blaming the victim. I realize if you do not have medical insurance, the emergency room, often, is the only place you can go for care. I am blaming our system that has created this waste of medical resources.

Medical providers are a large part of the problem that we see in today's emergency rooms. We, physicians, abuse this system. Because we are too busy, because we fear a medical malpractice suit or because we are too afraid of what we might encounter when we hear the details of certain medical cases, we too often send our patients to the emergency room, rather than see them ourselves. Do you want proof of this? Listen to the very first prompt the next time you call your doctor's office. It will say something like "If you are having a true medical emergency, please hang up and call 911." The message that is not so subtly conveyed to patients is that, "Don't even bother trying to get help from us, just go straight to the emergency room." And patients do. Throughout the rest of this book, I will discuss other ways that the proposed SPUN Health Insurance plan will discourage the unnecessary use of expensive emergency services. Starting with a significant co-pay for such service is the first.

As part of the fairness that should be built into any healthcare insurance plan, patients should not be penalized for under-calling what level of medical service they require. Under today's rules, if you go to your family doctor and she then sends you to a specialist for that problem, you have two co-pays, one for each of the two physicians you see. Or say you go to an urgent care center for an ankle injury and it is too serious for them to treat and they refer you to a regular emergency room. Again, you will incur two co-pays, one for each facility. Under my proposed SPUN plan, if you start out by going to a lower level of care and they cannot completely fix the problem, then the amount you paid for the first co-pay is credited toward the payment of the second, higher level of service. Following the above examples, that means you would only pay $25 (The $50 specialist fee co-pay minus $25 primary co-pay fee.) to see that specialist and $100 (The $200 emergency room co-pay minus $100 urgent care co-pay.) to go to the emergency room to have your injured ankle fixed.

In addition, under our SPUN plan, a co-pay would be waived if your acute problem is not solved, as long as you go back to the original facility. You should not to keep paying one if your problem does not improve. The logic behind this madness will accomplish several positive things for our healthcare system. First, patients are more likely to go back to the same physician that originally took care of them because there is no addition out of pocket cost for them. Obviously, this is most efficient in finding the answers to their medical problems and most efficient for the entire system in terms of dollars and cents. Second, there is a motivation for healthcare providers to spend time with the patient and get an answer the first time, as they lose the fee for co-payment every time a patient returns for the same problem. Third, by fixing medical problems more often on the first try, there will be less total return visits for the system, a further savings in total health expenditures. Obviously, the co-pay would not be waived if the patient has a chronic problem that requires on-going care.

The third and last out of pocket expense for us under this proposed SPUN plan would be for a few rare prescriptions and other pharmacologic costs. Not dissimilar what is seen today in most prescription plans, all medications would be categorized into one of three levels. At the base of our prescription plan under SPUN are medications that would be available at no cost to the patient. The list of base medications will include ones that can treat virtually every medical condition. For each condition, there would be several alternatives, if they exist, giving both practitioners and patients choices. This base list would contain both over the counter and prescription medications and generic and brand medications.

Why include non-prescription medications? Often, the over the counter medication is the least expensive and just as good as prescription ones. For example, over the counter prenatal vitamins are basically the same as much more expensive generic and brand prescription ones. Today, practitioners sometimes prescribe the prescription medications because the patient's co-payment may be less expensive than her cost for the over the counter. But it makes that cost more expensive for the entire system. By making over the counter medications part of the tier one, there are huge potential savings for the system, with no loss of efficacy.

The government, being the only entity in the country paying for medications, would have a huge hammer to use to drive down that nail of drug costs. It is no secret that the same medications, when sold in the United States cost more here than in in the rest of the world. This is even after "discounts" the manufacturers give, when selling them in the United States. It is why we, Americans, often go to Canada and Mexico to buy our medications. They are less expensive out of the country. This is in spite of the fact that so many medications are both developed and manufactured here. To use a non-medical analogy with you, it is as if Apple kept developing new models of iPhones and iPads in the United States but sold them for the highest price in our country with a discount for the rest of the world. It is interesting to note that even those of an "America First" political persuasion never raises this clear example of a policy that puts our country last.

Do want proof that medications cost more in the United States? Table 20 lists of some commonly prescribed medications and what they actually cost the patient in the United States compared with selected other countries in the world. The data comes from a Bloomberg News analysis of December 18, 2015.

Table 20. Cost of a Month's Supply of Selected Medications in Different Countries

Crestor (lipid lowering medication made by Astra Zeneca of the United Kingdom and Sweden)

Country	Cost
United States	$86.40
Germany	$40.50
Canada	$32.10
China	$32.00
Australia	$8.70
India	$3.60

Advair (asthma medication made by Glaxo Smith Kline of the United Kingdom)

Country	Cost
United States	$154.80
Canada	$74.12
Germany	$37.71
China	$32.00
Australia	$29.28
India	$10.12

Januvia (diabetes medication made by Merck of the United States)

Country	Cost
United States	$168.61
Canada	$68.10
Germany	$39.00
Australia	$33.60
China	$18.00
India	$13.80

Herceptin (breast cancer medication made by Roche of Switzerland)

Country	Cost
United States	$4,754.45
Canada	$3,546.87
Germany	$3,185.87
Australia	$3,141.84
China	$2,310.02
India	$2,196.44

Gleevec (chronic myeloid leukemia medication made by Novaris of Australia)

Country	Cost
United States	$10,122.30
Germany	$3,003.30
Australia	$2,585.10
Canada	$2,420.70

Notice for every medication listed, the cost to the patient was highest in the United States. It did not matter if the drug was developed by a company based here or not. Also, note that patients in other countries do not pay more for medications that are developed by *their* own companies.

Proof that Americans overpay for all medications, not just a few selected ones, comes from a CNN report of March 15, 2018. They found the per capita spending for drugs in the United States was more than $1,400 in 2016 while it was only $750 per person as an average for peer nations, a pool of countries that included Western Europe, Japan, Australia and Canada.

You may ask how much potential savings for healthcare in the United States is there if we were to bring down the amount we pay for medications to that of the rest of the world? Again, I like to be conservative in my estimations, though in my heart I know it could be much more than I calculated. First, let us assume that the cost of the above medications in the United States compared to the rest of the world represents the amount we overpay for all medications we buy. Second, then let us assume that we could only bring down the cost of medications to the second country's costs on our list. I do not think that is much of a stretch. Still, this means we would be paying only 47.9% as much on medications as we do now. Right now, we spend 14% of our health budget on medications. That may not seem a lot but remember our total annual medical budget is $3.3 trillion. Or put another way, we now spend $462 billion each year on medications. Therefore, our conservative cost for medications under our future SPUN plan would be 47.9% of that number or $221 billion. That represents a savings of $240 billion or 7% of our total medical expenses. If you do not want to implement any other change to our healthcare system, please agree with me to do this one. This is the low hanging fruit for us to pick. Let us have one national payer for our medications.

Why is medication cost so high in the United States? Much ink has been spilled and many bytes of data sent over the internet debating this question. Aaron Kesselheim and other researchers from the Harvard School of Medicine in 2016 looked at all the data from thousands of articles published over many years that studied the problem to reach a definitive answer. Funded by the Laura and John Arnold Foundation and the Engelberg Foundation, they published their conclusions in the medical journal JAMA in 2016. The number one reason for our high drug costs is that we do not have a national health insurance or similar program that can negotiate with the drug manufacturers for lower prices as is done in the rest of the world. We do not use our clout of numbers to bring down prices. You would expect a rental car company to be able to purchase its fleet of rental vehicles at a lower price than you or I when we buy our lone automobile. You would expect a restaurant to pay less for fruits and vegetables than you or I. But the opposite is true for our medications. We pay retail prices while the rest of the world pays wholesale.

Even when we had an opportunity to negotiate for lower medications prices, we failed to act. In 2003, Congress did a wonderful thing (Yes, it does happen, sometimes.) They passed a drug benefits bill for Medicare that finally gave seniors some relief in purchasing medications. However, they foolishly wasted that opportunity to try to get lower price for those medications. They were the Enterprise Rental Car Company paying sticker price for every one of a huge fleet of Ford cars.

The second reason medication costs are so high here compared with the rest of the world is now the patent system in our country works for the drug manufacturers rather than for the consumers. I am not saying we should not have a patent system to protect intellectual property. It makes sense that the United States has a system by which the developer of a new medicine has the exclusive rights to make and sell a medication for 20 years. After that time, other companies can make it. This is the origin of all the generic medications that are on the market. You say it is a fair system, right? After all, it encourages companies to do their research and development, knowing that in the end, they will make a profit off of their work. And after a time, the patent expires so then the cost of the medication will come down.

However, this system is abused. First, instead of trying to make truly new medications, drug manufacturers just slightly change an existing one and claim it a "new" medicine. That starts their 20-year timer over again, so they can sit back and collect more huge profits of an old drug. How do they pull this off? Tiny changes are made to dosages. A second truly non-therapeutic agent is added. The coating or delivery mechanism of the medication to the body is tweaked. A medication might be made in a chewable form rather than a pill or a capsule. An old medication is launched as an entirely new medication with a new name when it receives an indication to treat a new condition.

An example of this tiny change that results in a new

medication is what happened to the status of the inhalers used to treat asthma. Inhalers are small handheld devices that deliver asthma medication to the lungs of sufferers using a propellent. The propellent used to be chlorofluorocarbon (CFC). But that propellent, also used in air-conditioning, refrigerants and aerosol cans, was found to harm the ozone layer of the atmosphere. So, the Food and Drug Administration ordered CFC be removed from inhalers by 2008 and replaced by the propellant hydroflouroalkane (HFA) to help save the planet. The drug manufactures dutifully complied. Afterall, it was a windfall for them as essentially the same medications were considered new ones. The patent life was extended and the cost of a whole group of commonly used drugs increased threefold. (University of Florida. "New Asthma Inhaler Propellant Effective, But Costlier." ScienceDaily. www.sciencedaily.com/releases/2007/03/070329075220.htm)

The second problem with our drug patent system is that generic manufacturers are paid off by the original medication developer to delay the launch of their alternatives. Think of this as a legal bribe to eliminate the competition.

Third, the Food and Drug Administration (FDA), which must approve all drugs before they can be sold, is inefficient in approving generic medications. There often is a delay of three to four years before they reach the market. That represents three to four years that we all pay more for the brand medication.

Finally, certain present-day laws discourage the use of less expensive generics. For example, in over half the states, pharmacists are required to patient consult before switching a patient from a brand name to generic equivalent medication.

We must fix these loopholes in law or rather fix the huge gaps in the law that only serve to inflate pharmaceutic costs. Patents should not be issued for slight tweaks in a medication's formulation or new indications, only for true new drugs. The FDA should be much more efficient in approving generic medications. Laws should encourage the development and use of generics.

The third reason medications are so expensive in the United States is that a vast pharmaceutical-insurance-medical complex exists. It is not unlike the military-industrial complex President Eisenhower warned about in 1961, as he was about to leave office. He worried about the self-serving threat to our country of the tight union of the armed forces and defense contractors. The pharmaceutical-insurance-medical complex is a three-way union of the drug manufacturers, the administrators of medication benefits used by the medical insurance company and the medical providers.

They scratch each other's back. They serve each other more than they serve the patients. The pharmaceutical industry employs an army of salespeople to encourage physicians to prescribe their latest (and therefore, most expensive) medications. Is it fair that such a drug salesperson can barge into any doctor's office at any time and demand an audience with your physician, while you have a longer wait for an appointment you scheduled three months ago? The drug manufacturers make sweet deals with the medication benefits administrators that benefit the administrators, financially. more than lower the cost of medications to patients. Doctors yield to the pressure from free meals brought to their offices to feed their staffs by the drug companies and their high speaker fees for medical conferences to prescribe more costly medications. If we are to have lower drug prices, we must break up this pharmaceutical-insurance-medical complex that encourages the use of higher priced drugs, pushed by the manufacturers, encouraged by the benefit administrators and prescribed by the physicians, none of whom have to pay for them. Our tier system would break the power of this powerful complex.

How would the SPUN Health Insurance determine what medications would fall into this first, "no cost" tier? It will be modeled from two present day systems: one medical and one, non-medical. Today, hospitals and other larger purchasers of medications have formularies. A formulary is a tabulation of medications that are preferred lower cost ones used in the organization. It includes both prescription and over the counter medications. It includes both brand name and generic medications. The hospital or other organization has a committee to determine what medications make the list. The committee is made up by experts including physicians, pharmacists and other health professionals. It uses their combined expertise and considers such factors as safety, efficiency and cost. As new medications come to market, each are evaluated as to whether they will be added to the formulary. The formulary is a living creature, continually being reviewed and updated. A formulary is a beautiful thing for it has only a fraction of possible medications but can treat virtually any medical condition.

As a non-medical example, think of a potential SPUN formulary as your household's food shopping list. A budget conscious family will create a grocery list from all possible items at the food store that are available. It picks the ideas on the list out of consideration of cost and quality. The list covers all the major food groups but is contains only a tiny fraction of all the things that purchased at the store. It leans heavily on "generic" products, such as store brands, to save money. As new products come out, items may be added to the list or substituted for ones already on the grocery list. The grocery list is not completely rigid as sometimes the family will need to buy things not on the list.

Once the National Health Insurance committee has created its medication formulary, it will use a competitive bid process to determine which ones it will actually purchase. At first, it will put out feelers for bids from the pharmaceutic industry. The government is used to this model for purchasing. It is what is does when it buys anything it needs from toilet paper to guns.

The winning pharmaceutic products would be the lowest bidders in each medication category. Like it does today, the Food and Drug Administration would continue to monitor the manufacture and safety of the medications. The medications still would be sold in retail and on-line pharmacies. And they would get the medications form distributers who would get the medications from the manufacturers. As we shall see, there would be other outlets for medication sales, too. Only, the price would be fixed, determined by our competitive bid process. Again, this is no different than what the wise budget-conscious family does when they food shop. They use their grocery list and compare prices at several stores to get the best bargain for its food needs.

The pharmaceutical companies finally would become like any other company in the marketplace. They would be competing among themselves to make the best product in order to get on the formulary list and make that product at the lowest price to win in the competitive bidding process. It would be very competitive and worth their effort to do so as the National Health Insurance would be for all intents and purposes, the only buyer of medications in the country. This would have a dramatic impact on our medication costs, lowering them to that of the rest of the world.

Let us take as an example, oral contraceptives, so-called "birth control pills." There are between 100 and 200 brands on the market. As any gynecologist (myself, included) will tell you, they are all about the same. Each is made up of a synthetic estrogen and progestin, two different female hormones, in different formulations and dosage. Most of the variations are the same basic formulation. Most "new" brand oral contraceptives, too, are just slight rehashes of old formulations, created to give the manufacturer a new patent. The world does not need new forms of slightly rehashed oral contraceptives, which the present system seems to encourage. What it needs are entirely new contraceptive methods. Under the proposed SPUN Health

Insurance program, a committee would decide on just two dozen or so oral contraceptives for its formulary. Then, competitive bids would go out to the manufacturers, resulting in about a dozen that would be covered for sale without a cost to the user. Because the process would be so competitive, this would result in low cost oral contraceptives for the system, no cost for the women who use it and fewer unwanted pregnancies (the goal for using the product and better for society). It also would discourage pharmaceutical companies from reinventing the wheel and just rebranding old products but would encourage them to research entirely new forms of contraception.

What if a physician and patient decide it would be best to use a medication that did not make the cut for the competitive bid process. Such medications still would be covered by the National Health Insurance, but the patient would have to pay the extra cost difference of the medication versus the one on the formulary. Continuing our oral contractive example, let us say a patient and her gynecologist decide that Brand Q oral contraceptive would be best for her, but Brand Q is not covered but is on the formulary. Brand Q costs $50 for a month supply. The brand on the formulary costs $35 a month. The patient would be responsible for the difference of $15 for each month. Brand Q and medications like it would be "tier two" formulations under the health plan.

What if the medication is not on the formulary at all? Medications that did not make the "cut" would be ones that have been shown to be ineffective, expensive, replaced by better alternatives or dangerous. These medications would not be covered at all under the National Health Insurance plan and the patient would have to pay the full cost. These would be the "tier three" drugs.

That would be it for all the expenses that we would be expected to pay under the SPUN Insurance Plan. To summarize, we would pay for certain non-covered, elective medical procedures, reasonable, tiered for level of service co-pays, and some unusual medication costs. The plan would have a reward or payment plan to the patient, too. This is to encourage us to be stay and get healthy. Americans, compared with people in other developed countries, have a lot of bad health habits. We do not eat right, exercise enough, get the preventative care that we need and follow up with care when we should. These habits are particularly bad among the poor. As a society in general and as part of the SPUN Health Plan, in particular, we need to encourage good health behaviors. This will have a twofold benefit for our society. We will be healthier, and it will save the healthcare system money. This reward system that is so unique to this plan has a whole chapter to itself, the next one of this book.

Today, it seems that medical care for certain parts of your body are not as necessary as other parts. Your teeth, for example, are not covered by your general medical plan. You need a separate dental plan, with its own rules and regulations. The same thing goes for eye care. Are not eating and seeing just as important as any other health concern? Why do we have to carry yet another card around and deal with yet another medical insurance company and its bureaucracy for certain parts of our body?

The third aspect of our proposed National Health Insurance plan is that there is just one medical plan for your whole body! It is silly that today there are separate medical insurance plans for your general health, for your teeth, for your eyes, for mental health, for your medications and for long term care insurance. Because the simplest plan usually is the best, having one plan will make it easier for both patients and providers. (It starts with having to just carry one health insurance card around with you!) Merging all the insurances together will save the system money, too as patients and providers will not waste time determining which of the smaller plans is the one that is covering a particular illness.

Mental health, although part of most present medical plans, usually has different rules compared with the rest of the insurance plan. Coverage is skimpier and harder to get. It is as if to say depression is not as serious disease as diabetes or bipolar disorder not as important to recognize and treat as heart disease. Shame on us for perpetuating that kind of thinking today. It is a prejudice as significant as occurs against minorities, women and people with different sexual orientation. According to the National Mental Health Foundation, 43.8 million of us will have mental illness in a given year. That is one in five Americans. Ten million, or one in 25, will have a serious mental disorder. The scope of the individual diseases also is staggering. There are 2.4 million Americans with schizophrenia, 6.1 million with bipolar disorder, 16 million suffer with major depression and 42 million have an anxiety disorder.

There is no better example than the behavioral health fields of what we do, proactively, as a society about our health that will influence so many other aspects of how we live. Better mental health means a better society. It is much more than the rash of mass shootings that we have witnessed in recent years. Look at our opioid abuse epidemic. Mental health and addiction disorders are often linked. About 10.2 million Americans suffer from both mental health disorder and drug addiction. About one quarter of our adult homeless population have a severe mental health disease. The same statistic holds true for our prison population. Ninety percent of suicide victims had underlying mental illness. Removing the obstacles to and aggressively recognizing and treating mental illness will make us a better and happier people.

I know. I know. I hear you. You say we can't afford to pay for such treatment. I say, we cannot afford not to pay for treating mental illness. For example, depression is the number one cause of disability in the world. In the United States, alone, $193 billion is lost in earnings from severe mental illness.

Today, instead of doing everything we can to treat these diseases, we put up barriers. Only 40% of adults with mental illness received treatment of any kind in the last year. That number is only 50% for children between ages 8 and 15 years. Why do they not get the treatment they need? Lack of medical insurance for mental health services is a huge barrier. A study by the Center for Disease Control found that in 2014, 9.5% of Americans with severe mental illness did not have insurance that covered seeing a psychiatrist or counselor. Furthermore, 10.5% had delays in getting treatment because of "insurance issues" and 10% could not afford their medications for their disorders.

Like so many things in American medicine, small cracks in the system are caught in a positive feedback loop leading to giant canyons. Because the system pays so poorly for mental health services, not enough bright people go into the field. Psychiatrists rank near or at the bottom of the pay scale for physicians. Why would you go to medical school and become a psychiatrist when you can earn much more money being a plastic surgeon? This has created a shortage of behavioral health professionals, especially psychiatrists, nationwide. The problem is particularly acute in rural parts of the country. The solution is so simple. Basic economics says to cure a shortage increase the price for the service being provided. By covering and paying mental health professionals the same as other medical professionals, we would go a long way to making our country's mental health better and us a more productive society.

The plan also will eliminate the need for injury coverage for auto accidents and for workplace injuries. If you break your arm at work or are hurt in a car crash, the SPUN Health Insurance will pay for it. Think how much less expensive your car insurance will be! Businesses will save money, too, as a result, not having to purchase workman's insurance. Wait a second, you may say. Won't that just transfer the cost from the auto and workers insurance to the government? Yes, but the *total* cost to the country will be less. Much of the money that is paid for these insurances is for legal fees and other bureaucratic expenses as the injured and insurer duke it out, trying to figure out if an injury is due the car accident or due to the injury at the workplace.

The fourth tenet of the SPUN plan coverage is that all medical services that have a rational basis for being used will be covered by the plan. And if there is an uncertainty as to the efficiency of the treatment, the services will be covered until proven otherwise. How would the SPUN system decide if a given medical service is beneficial or not? Groups of experts from the given branch of medicine would decide and create guidelines. Cardiologists would decide what therapies are best for heart disease, for example. Such a system already exists but on a more informal level. Specialty groups put out bulletins that are continually being updated on what is safe and works and what is dangerous and does not work for the different medical conditions that they treat. On a larger scale, there are organizations like Cochrane. It is a non-profit organization that was formed in England about 25 years ago to answer such questions. It has 53 medical review groups and 30,000 volunteer experts from around the world which determine which diagnostic tests and treatments work, and which do not.

You ask how the various medical specialty groups will decide on what treatments are beneficial and what are not. I answer, simply. They will use science. They will review the medical studies that have been done in the past. That is the methodology of groups like Cochrane uses, today. Not all the medical data is equal and of course, some studies are better than others. The best information comes from what are called randomized control trials. With such studies, a question is asked, two groups are created which are as close to each other in characteristics as possible. This initial process is called randomization. Then one group has the test done or treatment performed, and the other does not. The first group is the treatment group. The second is the control group. Then, the two groups are followed up to see if there is a difference in outcome. If there is and the statistics bear it out, it can be concluded that the therapy works.

Let me give you a silly example of a randomized study and how it is done. Say you wanted to find out if a cookie will make you happy at work in the afternoon. (I think you know the answer to this already without the study.) To answer this question, you would create two groups of workers. Several measures would be taken to make sure the two groups are very similar to each other. That they have the same number of men and women, that similar age groups would be included, and that similar occupations tested. The test would be carried out on the same day of the week and same time of the year. The groups would have to include similar numbers of people with depression. Their general happiness and outlook on life should be very close to each other. This is not an easy task and the hardest part of most randomized control studies is the randomization. Then one group, the treatment group, would receive the treatment, a cookie and one would not, the control group. Then both groups would be interviewed or receive a questionnaire to see how happy they are, afterward. If the group that received a cookie was happier afterward and the statistics bear it out, then we can conclude that a cookie at work in the afternoon will make us happy.

You may be surprised to find that for most questions in medicine, truly excellent randomized control studies do not exist. Therefore, we must look to lower level studies. One such type is the retrospective study. It takes two groups of people, after the fact, each with a different outcome and looks back to see if there was a common cause to that result. The reason that these retrospective studies are not as reliable as randomized control studies is because human memory and human bias are such powerful influences.

Let us explore such an example of a retrospective study using the question that was posed about cookies and happiness. First, we find two groups of people, one happy and one not. Then we ask both groups if they had a cookie at work that day. If more of the people in the "happy group" had a cookie compared with the "unhappy group," then we can conclude that a cookie at work makes us happy. Can you see the problem is this study? Generally, more grumpy people are more likely to forget that they got a cookie at work and generally happier people are more likely to remember having a cookie, biasing the study's results.

Sometimes in medicine even retrospective studies do not exist. Then we must rely on the results of a single case or a small group of several reported cases. Continuing to follow our cookie study example, we would rely on the single observation that Joe was very happy after he received a free cookie at work and conclude everyone would benefit from that cookie. It is better than nothing. But the problem with such studies is that Joe could have been happier for many reasons other than the cookie or Joe might be unusually fond of cookies. It is making a giant leap from a single observation.

At the bottom of the medical data pyramid are expert opinions for even single case studies do not exist. All what we know about the best approach to a medical problem is based on their hunches and experiences. In our example case, we would ask the Cookie Monster of Sesame Street or Mrs. Fields if a cookie at work in the afternoon will make you happier. These "educated guesses" often are wrong. But physicians must act and work with what knowledge they have, even if they are working in the dark. For this might be the only course of action until better data comes along.

Regardless of our level of reliability, our proposed SPUN Health Insurance expert-generated guidelines would serve several purposes. Primarily, it would determine what medical tests and services would be covered by the plan and what would not. But it would go much further than that. It would be a wonderful reference and educational summary source of information for medical providers and patients as to the latest and best treatments. Also, it would identify what gaps there are in today's medical knowledge, stimulating tomorrow's research. Finally, it would be a two-way street, receiving all that medical data about the best course of action from the results from all of our treatments stored in the system. Later in this book, we will talk about this golden opportunity of data mining in medicine. For having a single payer system where everyone is receiving similar care means there will be more cumulative data that can be used to answer so many of the unanswered questions in medicine.

How would the patient and the medical provider know that the proposed diagnosis and treatment plan will be covered under the SPUN Plan? Instead of the present complex, expensive and frustrating pre-authorization process that exists, today, the approval would be determined in microseconds. The software built into the universal SPUN Plan electronic medical records would generate an answer, immediately. All the software would have to do is make sure that the test or treatment ordered for the diagnosis matches an approved one in the National Health Insurance database.

What happens when a patient and her physician decide on a therapy that is not typically covered by the plan? Sometimes, an experimental or non-conventional approach to a medical problem is best one. This will be the only time pre-authorization, so common today, would be needed. Right at the office visit, the physician and patient will contact an independent expert not directly employed by the SPUN Health Insurance service but available for such consultation. By being independent, the expert will not feel the pressure to save the system money but only to do the right thing by the patient. This can be done by an on-line chat directly from the universal electronic medical records. The expert will be a physician or similar professional in real world practice, who has experience in the condition that is being treated. She will have instant access to the medical records, making the determination faster and easier, and can talk directly to the patient and practitioner. She will be empowered to decide in an instant whether to approve the approach or not. If at the end of this group discussion, there was no agreement among the parties, there would be an appeal process available to ensure the patient's rights to unconventional care.

This leads us to the fifth aspect of the SPUN Plan coverage. It will cover many forms of non-traditional treatments and therapies. By non-traditional, I mean both alternative treatments which are used in place of conventional medicine and complementary medicine which is used alongside it. This is not a trivial consideration as over one third of Americans use at least one form of non-traditional medicine, annually.

What are the most commonly used non-traditional methods, today? There is acupressure where practitioners place pressure to specific points along the body's meridians. It is related to a second method, acupuncture, where specific points of the body are stimulated usually by needles or electrical stimulation. Third is aromatherapy, using oils extracted from plants, inhaled or rubbed into the skin to promote healing. Ayurveda is an ancient medical practice from India that uses a combination of herbs, message and diet. Hydrotherapy, also called balneotherapy, uses water to treat disease states. The practice includes such treatments as mudpacks, wraps and douches. Biofeedback therapies allow patients to control normally involuntarily bodily processes, such as heart rate, blood pressure, body temperature and muscle tension. Chiropractic medicine treats diseases of the bones, muscles and nervous system by spinal manipulation. Homeopathy uses extremely tiny doses of medicine to treat disease. Naturopathy uses the healing power of nature and is a combination of nutrition, behavioral changes, herbal medicine and homeopathy. Reflexology is the medical art of applying pressure to specific areas of the feet, hands and ears that are believed to correspond to certain body organs to improve their function. Finally, there is Reiki which believes illness means one's life energy is low, but it can be increased by transferring it from the practitioner to the patient using light touch.

These treatments, by definition, are highly controversial as to their efficacy. Most do not work any better than the placebo effect. However, some are effective. We should not dismiss out of hand all non-traditional therapies, but our system should not waste money on ineffective ones and even more importantly, delay effective treatment. The solution is simple as to which ones to cover. Just like for traditional medicine, let our experts comb the medical literature and find out to the best of our present-day knowledge what alternative medicine therapies work and what do not. Those that do work would then be the ones covered under the SPUN Health Insurance. That is not enough. The experts will create studies to test any gray areas of alternative medicine where the data is not yet clear. With the huge number of potential patients, it would be easy to do the medical research into their alternative therapies. With one insurance system, one set of medical records, one huge database, our SPUN Health Insurance has the potential to be the best medical research tool in the world.

We know some really basic measures, outside of traditional medicine, do work. The best examples are diet and exercise, like your mother told you when you were a child, protesting that bronchi on your dinner plate. What can the proposed National Health Insurance program do to encourage these basic health habits. What can our program do to motivate us to do our health maintenance? This is the subject of the next chapter as we detail how the program can incentivize us to be healthy.

5. HOW WILL SPUN MAKE US HEALTHIER?

My son, Matt, is a world champion blood donor. He gives blood at work every chance he can, usually every two months. As a retired physician, I admire his altruism, knowing how truly lifesaving blood can be and how often it is in short supply. I practiced obstetrics which unfortunately can be a "bloody business" and know the need for blood transfusions in this field is critical. But the cynical side of me also knows a second reason why he donates blood. He gets paid time off from work, every time he donates. What a wonderful system his company has! We all need a nice kick in the pants sometimes to do the right thing.

It is no secret that as a group, Americans are overweight, have a less than ideal diet, and do not exercise enough. For example, it is shocking when you travel to Europe to see there is lower incidence of obesity and the population generally is more activity. Correcting these basic problems of how we live will have many positive outcomes. Of course, it will make us all, healthier. It will save our SPUN Health Insurance system money taking care of medical problems caused by our poor lifestyle choices. We will be a more productive society, too, with less days and income lost from the illnesses that are the result of our unhealthy diets and lack of exercise.

Let us start with the problems with our diets. Over one-third of Americans are obese. It starts at a young age with 17% of children aged 2 to 19 years being obese. The lower the socioeconomic group you are in this country, the more likely you will be obese. Since the beginning of history, the poor were starved. It is ironic, today, thanks to unhealthy diets, obesity and poverty are strongly correlated. We, as a society, have a culture of cheap, fast, high calorie, low nutrition food. Part of the problem is that healthy fresh fruits and vegetables are relatively expensive. The problem starts before we are born as studies show what mothers eat during pregnancy influences both the choices their children make after they are born and influences their risk of obesity and diabetes.

Why is obesity such a big deal? It soon will be the number one cause of preventable deaths in our country, passing those caused by tobacco. Today, about 300,000 deaths, annually, in the United States are due to the effects of obesity. It is no different that each year all the people in a city the size of Tampa, Florida are erased off the map. What a human tragedy of enormous scale that is just not recognized! Not only does obesity increase the risk of heart disease and diabetes, but only increases the risk of certain cancers like that of the colon and breast. Obesity makes us less health in non-fatal ways, too. It affects our mobility and is a major contributor to degeneration of our bones and joints.

How do we get people to eat healthier foods? How do we influence their choices? Two ways: avoidance and cost. Let us tackle avoidance, first. If you wanted to improve your diet, you would make sure there were no cookies and potato chips in your cupboard. The government, at every level, should do the same thing. At every opportunity, it should try to take junk food away from us. They can make it harder for us to eat poorly. For example, many public school districts have taken the step of eliminating soda machines from the school grounds and junk food from the school cafeterias. Let us expand on this concept all across our society.

For example, any government-sponsored food program should not include unhealthy food. There are dozens of such programs, large and small, that have the admirable goal of relieving hunger by providing reduced cost or free food to the poor. The largest such program is called SNAP, short for the Supplemental Nutrition Assistance Program. Because in the past, purchases were made with them, SNAP still is called "food stamps." It provides direct financial assistance to buy food almost anywhere for those of us who are poor. I see an opportunity with SNAP for a positive health intervention. Today, unfortunately, there are very few restrictions as to what the recipients can purchase. These include alcohol, tobacco, hot and prepared foods to go, restaurant food and nonfood items. But there are no restrictions as to the quality of the food received from the program.

This is a missed opportunity to influence the health of Americans through their diet. And it would influence those who need the dietary help the most, the poor. SNAP and other government sponsored programs should not cover the purchase of junk foods. The usual response as to why junk foods are not excluded from such plans is that it would be too burdensome to identify what defines junk food. To that I answer, "cheese puffs!!!" Both defining and enforcing such a list of unhealthy foods would not be not difficult.

In 1964, the United States Supreme Court Justice Potter Stewart famously defined obscenity with the statement: "I know it when I see it!" The same holds true for junk food. Mmm. Potato chips, yes. Broccoli, no. But we can make it easier for government programs to decide whether a food is unhealthy or not. Already food labels have nutritional information on them. The gobs of data on such labels are helpful, but we need a simple system that interprets the data for all for us, including the government. One such system is used in Britain. It uses a stoplight symbolism for five food contents. "Green" means good, "yellow" means caution and "red" means stop and avoid. The five components of food analyzed with this system are total calories, sugar, total fat, saturated fat and salt. The coding standardizes the portion size, too, at 100 grams. To this symbolism, I would add an additional sixth summary stoplight in one of the three colors. Junk foods, high in concentrated calories, sugar, fat, saturated fat or salt would have a big red stop sign. Red stop sign foods will not be covered under any government food program.

We can do more than just not pay for junk food under governmental programs. We can tax them, too. This addresses the second cost factor that can influence our food choices. Any junk food with a total red stoplight label would have a significant tax of 50% added on it at time of purchase. For example, a $3 bag of potato chips would cost $4.50. Expense would be a powerful motivator to discourage their purchase, especially among the poor, who need all the help they can get to eat right. A few cities, like my hometown of Philadelphia, already have a similar beverage tax on soft drinks. To be truly effective, to motivate us all to consume less unhealthy food, the tax should cover *all* junk food and be *national*.

I am sure there would be much grumbling about such a tax. There would be anger about the cost burden that will place on us, the imposition on our freedom to kill ourselves with our forks. My answer is that government has an obligation to use its taxing power to discourage activities that are not good for us. Plus, we already have such a system in place, just on a much smaller scale. Today, there are significant taxes on booze and cigarettes. It is Economics 101 that higher prices lower demand. Let us take advantage of Adam Smith's laws to lower our risk of the soon to be number one preventable cause of death in our country, obesity.

The SPUN System food tax would include a carrot (pun

intended) as well as a stick. Healthy foods, the green light ones, would be subsidized by the tax collected on the red-light foods. As we have seen, a significant reason that the poor do not consume enough fresh fruits and vegetables is their high cost. Just like a higher price decreases demand, a lower price will increase it. Why buy a $4.50 bag of chips when you can purchase a fifty cent one-pound bag of fresh apples?

How can our National Health Insurance program get us to exercise more, move more in general, get off the couch and look away from our cellphone screens? At a minimum, the system will cover the cost of a basic gym memberships. It will be covered only if it is being used. Therefore, if you join a fitness club but do not use it, you will not be reimbursed for the cost of it. The problem with most gym memberships is that people often join them, for example, as part of a New Year's resolution. Then, soon, by Ground Hog's Day, the motivation is gone, and they stop going. One way is to keep people going to the gym is for the SPUN Health Insurance to only reimburse the cost of the membership after the participant has gone a certain number of times per year, for example one hundred

Federal business tax law can be changed as part of SPUN to encourage gyms at the workplace. Making it easier and more convenient to use the gym will be another potent motivator. On a larger scale, the government should do more to encourage us to move our butts. We should build more playgrounds in the cities and have more organized activities. That is because the poor in the city, today, have less access to recreational facilities. These are needed for children who at the highest risk of developing sedentary life styles. These playgrounds need to be developed, made safe and accessible, staffed and offer a variety of activities for people of all ages.

Our infrastructure must change. It is relatively easy to add more bike lanes. In cities, there should be bike racks everywhere. Bicycle share programs are wonderful and can be expanded.

There needs to be more walking trails and planned communities that are pedestrian friendly. Even improving our train and mass transportation infrastructure would help. These forms of transportation involve more walking compared to cars, as well as being better for our environment.

A basic tenet of our future healthcare plan is that it should include more than the prevention, diagnosis and treatment of disease. It should be part of a new philosophy for our society. It should become part of our national fabric that we are an active, outdoor-orientated, nature-loving, healthy-eating people. For us to change our behaviors, we must change our way of thinking. All levels of government and all parts of society must be involved in this effort. From school districts to large corporations, from city planners to youth church groups, we, all, must think differently so our children can live as long, productive and healthy lives as we are.

How else, besides improving our diet and activity levels can the SPUN Health Insurance program encourage us to be healthy? "Opting out" versus "opting in" health strategies are yet another way. Let us explore the frequently cited example of "opting out," organ donation. Everyone agrees that organ donation is life-saving, but the technology is limited by the number of donor organs. Now, most states, as part of the driving license process, ask you if you want to be an organ donor. The default choice is not to be one. This is an "opt in" system and it is what we are used to seeing for most volunteer programs. A better strategy, according to modern economists, would be an "opt out" one. When one's driver's license is renewed, automatically make everyone a potential organ donor. If someone has personal or religious objection to being a potential organ donor, then they can make the choice not to be one. Spain, today, has such a system, and not surprisingly, the country has the highest organ donor rates in the world.

The idea is signing people up for positive health

111

interventions automatically, rather than overcoming their inertia of doing the leg work. The "opt out" system has worked for diabetes interventional behavioral programs, getting patients to do randomized control medical studies, and in HIV testing. Our SPUN Health Insurance program can encourage further use of "opt out" healthcare by providing the necessary legal framework for it.

What would be potential areas of healthcare that would benefit from such an "opt out" system? Besides registering everyone as a potential organ donor, we can have a jury duty system of blood donation. Blood donation is another critical area where there are many potential donors, but few actually participate. Like being called for jury duty, if there is a need for blood donors, the SPUN Health System can recruit donors by snail mail or e-mail with a scheduled time and place for the donation. Like for jury duty, employers would have to honor the request and pay the employee for the time they would miss work. The donor would get a small allowance, "jury duty pay" for their time and trouble. Potential blood donors who have a religious, personal, or medical reason not to give blood, of course, could opt out. Though many people would opt out, enough potential donors could be recruited to maintain society's supply of blood without the struggles we see today. I believe people are inherently good, but we just can be a bit lazy and need a kickstart to do the right thing.

Medical providers should have automatic scheduling of future screening and follow-up appointments for their services and those already in place should be better utilized. My dentist has his patients schedule their next cleaning and check up at the current one. His philosophy is that no one wants to go to the dentist and it becomes easy to "forget" to schedule your next appointment. Having a future visit scheduled overcomes this inertia. Our present medical system can do much more to ensure patients get both preventative and follow up care.

Our present medical appointment scheduling system is a nightmare. It is easier to book a trip around the world than schedule a medical test or a visit at a new practice. Although some practices have on line scheduling of appointments, most still do it as was done in 1960, by telephone. It is slow, inefficient and expensive. No one wants to deal with overworked, often rude medical schedulers. The thought of yet again confronting all the insurance and personal questions is a major roadblock to us getting our care. So, we don't. Later in this book we will detail our plan for a universal system of medical records and software. Part of it though, will be on line scheduling. If Open Table can book a restaurant reservation for us anywhere in the world, our SPUN Health Insurance should be able to schedule a screening mammogram at our local hospital. Since the system will know all your personal details already, and there is only one insurance plan, there will be no need for all the repetition of the same questions. Providers also will have access to the system, so they can schedule not only visits with their own practice but with any other in the country. For example, when you go to the gynecologist for your annual examination, your mammography can be scheduled for you as you check out. Having the appointment in the book will encourage us to do what we know that we should do but often do not want to do.

The system should encourage physicians and other medical providers to do as much as possible at a single visit. If a patient comes in for a problem and they happen to be due for routine care, that should be performed at the same time. Likewise, if a problem is found during a check-up, the evaluation should begin at once. The less hurdles there are for medical care, the more likely it will be performed. It is just common sense. Today, the insurance system often discourages such "bundling of care." Providers often do not get paid for anything extra they do at a patient encounter. We should be doing the opposite. Let us streamline the number of encounters as much as possible. We get the care we deserve. We lose less time from work and from the rest of our lives, making us a more efficient as well as a healthier society. It saves the healthcare system money in the long run as there are fewer total encounters for registering, billing and paperwork.

Continuing this theme of using "opt out" medical services. the SPUN Health Insurance system will have incentives for health practices that have vertical rather than horizontal integration. Today, many medical practices are huge corporations of a dozen or more physicians with a huge supporting staff. The sign on their doors with the practitioners' names look like that of a law firm. Of course, there is something to be said for a larger size as there are efficiencies to be gained. But almost all these large practices are of the *same* medical specialty. There are large groups of cardiologists and large groups of urologists and large groups of orthopedic surgeons. In business, they call this approach, horizontal integration. This is increasing the number of widget makers at the same level of production. What is needed in modern medicine is vertical integration, that is, combining widget makers and doohickey makers and thingamajig makers under the same umbrella.

You may ask what the advantage is of combining different specialties in the same practice. Patients can move seamlessly between physicians when they have a problem that bridges more than one specialty. Let us take a simple example. A woman over 40 years old comes in for a routine gynecologist examination. As part of the consultation, she is going to receive a prescription for a screening mammography for detecting early breast cancer. In most cases, today, she is going to have to go to another facility. You know what that means to have that test. That means, calling that facility, choosing from a bewildering selection from the phone tree, waiting on hold for a receptionist to answer her call, negotiating with the receptionist for an appointment, answering the same dozen or so questions about insurance and other personal information and waiting for that appointment. So many obstacles can occur before that appointment. She may forget, get sick or just cancel it because, let us face it, no woman really wants to have a mammography. It also involves taking another day or part day off from work or getting a babysitter. Then, she must travel to the facility, go through the bureaucracy of registration, then the wait for her appointment. All before actually having the test performed. Not only is all this inefficient, costing the medical care system the costs of arranging for two visits, it costs society even more in the lost productivity of this patient. Since we know in advance what we are going to have to go through, each added step in the process means an opportunity for us to just chuck it and not go.

This is a very simple and common example. Often, a patient's problem involves a half dozen or more different medical provider entities. That includes the medical laboratory for blood testing, radiology, different specialists and pharmacy visits. Each requires separate appointments. Each requires scheduling, bureaucracy and waiting. Each represents a series of roadblocks for us to just give up, turn around and not get the care we need. In a later chapter, we will talk more about the process of vertical integration in providing healthcare and how our SPUN Health Insurance plan can make it happen. Suffice for now to say it is an important component of the "opt out" thinking, our medical system needs.

Part of our thinking about medical care must change. The sooner we can take care of a problem, the more effective the treatment will be. Not only is it more effective, it is less expensive, too. This is common sense. It is less expensive to repair a roof than replace it. That is why it is so important to fundamentally change how we as Americans live. Our diets. Our activities. Our lifestyles. Just as important is preventative care and health screening. It is funny that we live in a world where our cars must undergo inspection every year as required by the state department of motor vehicles, but there is no such requirement for our bodies.

How else can the SPUN Health Insurance encourage us towards preventive medicine? I believe money talks. Instead of us paying for the services, or even not charging us out of pocket for such preventive services, the system should *pay us* to do healthy things. Money talks! It is motivating for everyone, but it particularly would be motivating to the poor. By definition, they could use the funds, the most. Also, they are the ones most likely not to do such preventive measures. I believe by paying patients for preventative care, in the long run it will save the system money by disease prevention and early detection.

The dollar amount of the patient prevention payment would be in proportion to the unpleasantness of the task and the effort it takes to complete it. For example, routine physicals, annual eye examinations, annual flu shots and other standard immunizations would pay a modest $25.

Including immunizations is critical to the plan. As we have seen in the first chapter, Americans have one of the lowest immunization rates in the world. Part of this is based on pseudo-science and fear mongering misinformation. But most of it is pure inertia. Because it is so hard to deal with our broken healthcare system, it discourages even the simplest of health tasks, like immunizations. Changing the whole fabric of the system to make it user friendly and giving financial incentives can overcome this inertia. Most times when you take a positive step for your health, whether you get a mammogram or lose excessive weight, it just benefits you. For immunizations, it benefits everyone in society when you get that shot. This is because of the concept of herd immunity. Most immunizations are not 100% effective in preventing an infectious disease. But the more people who get inoculated, the less chance there will be for someone to pass on the disease to someone else. Your influenza shot protects both you and me from getting the flu.

More unpleasant health tasks would reward you $50. These would include gynecological examinations, mammograms and dental checkups. Tasks that patients really avoid would pay $100. The best example of this is colonoscopy. From my years of practice, I discovered almost all patients over age 45 years know they should have a colonoscopy for early prevention and detection of colon polyps and cancers. They agree it was an important test, but fear of the preparations for the tests (all the laxatives) and the sedation for the test, itself, is a roadblock for them to actually have the test. There also is what I call the "yuck factor." Because the test *sounds* so unpleasant, why would I want to do it? But when patients who finally underwent the procedure, most were surprised how not so unpleasant it was, after all and would do it again. To overcome patients' fears and the "yuck factor," let us pay them. If it works for all those people on reality TV shows to do unpleasant things for money, why not for our health?

Another example of a "big payday" for screening would be testing that requires multiple visits. For example, prenatal care typically requires a dozen or so office visits during a woman's pregnancy. That such care leads to healthier mothers and babies is an established fact. It is cost effective, too. It is estimated that a dollar spent on prenatal care saves the healthcare system $8 later, But, especially among the poor, prenatal care is spotty, at best. Therefore, let us pay pregnant women $100 if they make all of their prenatal visits.

The payment system also would extend to patients with chronic diseases to motivate them to get the necessary follow up testing. Let us take the example of adults with Type II diabetes. Such patients are at much higher risk of heart and other cardiovascular disease, retinal eye disease, kidney disease and foot disease. They need screening for both how well their blood sugars are being controlled and for all the possible complications of their diabetes. Compliance is notoriously poor. Let the SPUN

National Health System pay them $100 if they complete all of their screening tests each year.

Let us go a step further. Let the SPUN system pay diabetic patients if they lower and maintain lower blood sugars. How well a diabetic patient keeps his blood sugars in check can be determined using a simple blood test, called a hemoglobin A1c. It measures the average blood sugar over the past three months. It is the most important number for a diabetic as the higher the hemoglobin A1c, the greater the chance for the serious complications of diabetes. To motivate Type II diabetic patients, let us pay them $500 for each drop in their hemoglobin A1c value toward the normal range, and if they lower and maintain a lower number for two consecutive three-month measures in a row. The motivation would be voluntary but double-edged. If the hemoglobin A1c went up, the patient would have to pay back the reward.

There are many chronic medical conditions that have the potential for a voluntary, monetary reward system. Think hypertension and weight loss. We must think outside of the box and try new ways of attacking the roots of our national sickness. Too much of our future is at stake is keep ignoring it.

6. HOW WILL MEDICAL PROVIDERS GET PAID?

We all expect to be paid fairly for our work and pay fairly for work done for us. The same should be true about our medical care. We want to pay fairly for our healthcare services, even if we are not directly paying for it. Because after all, it is coming out of our pockets in the long run, regardless of the payment scheme.

Before we start our proposals for payment under the SPUN Healthcare Plan, we must get back to basics. We must understand the different ways that we can get paid and can pay other people. It matters because of our human nature. Let us start with a simple example. If you have children at home, think about the different ways you can pay them for doing their chores. Take, for example, having your son or daughter rake the fall leaves in the backyard. There are three different systems you could use. You could pay them by the task. That is, give them a set amount for the entire chore. Second, you could pay them hourly, by the number of hours they work. Or finally, you could create a metric that judges how well they did the chore. They will try to "work" the payment system, no matter which one you choose. This is not to say your children are diabolic, just human.

If you pay them by the chore, they will be motivated to complete the entire task, quickly as possible. But they may rush a little too fast through the chore, leaving many leaves behind, just to get finished and paid. If you pay them by the hour, they will be more compulsive, knowing the longer they work the more money they earn. But they will be more inefficient in the task, taking longer than needed. Finally, if you pay them based on a set parameter, like the numbers of leaves remaining under a certain tree, they will tend to address just that parameter, ignoring the overall condition of the yard, to maximize their profits. With this third payment system, there will be a lot more discussion between you and your child as to how well they met the parameter that you chose to pay them.

In the adult world, we almost always use the first or second payment system for services we use. When we have a plumber fix a broken pipe in our house, we will either pay a set amount for the repair or pay them by the hour. Most workers are either salaried employees, which is a way of getting paid by the task or hourly employees, payment based on time. For example, teachers are salaried, getting a set pay, regardless of the number of hours they work. Fast food restaurant employees and lawyers, obviously two very different careers, are hourly, getting paid by the number of hours they work.

Let us turn to healthcare. How are medical providers, such as physicians, healthcare workers and hospitals paid today? All three methods of payment are used. For example, medical procedures, like surgeries and dental work, are paid by the task. If a surgeon removes your gallbladder, the medical insurance company will pay her a set fee for all the care related to the surgery, from the time of making the diagnosis and consultation in the office, through surgery and hospital care afterward, to postoperative follow-up care back in the office. Insurance companies will pay a set fee to an outpatient clinical laboratory or hospital or other facility performing a blood test for cholesterol on a covered patient. The advantage of by paying by the task is that is makes medical procedures more efficient. Remember it is just human nature. If you are paying by the task, you will motivate people to complete the task as quickly and efficiently as possible. That is why surgeons always seem in a hurry! It also is why most blood tests in the country are performed at huge national clinical laboratories to take advantage of the economy of scales. Unfortunately, paying by the task has a downside. It means skimping on the quality. It is why you will rarely get more than a two-minute conversation with most surgeons. It is why your visits to outpatient clinical laboratory centers feel like McDonald's at lunchtime, but without the French fries.

Physicians, when they are not doing procedures like surgery, are paid for their ability to diagnosis disease and create a plan for treatment. The traditional way physicians are paid is fee for service. On the surface, this, too, is getting paid by task. Each office, hospital or emergency room encounter is charged a certain amount of money to the insurance company. As we saw earlier in this book, the insurance company, along with the out of pocket cost paid by the patient, pays a much smaller, contracted, set amount of this bill.

Obviously, it takes more time, effort and experience to evaluate and treat a couple with years of infertility than an uncomplicated urinary tract infection. Can you recognize, too, that some cases of infertility are easier to cure than others and the same goes for bladder infections? How does the present payment system compensate for the differences in work that the physician must do in these different cases? It uses our last method, payment by formula. It is time for a strong cup of coffee, dear reader, as we reenter the strange and illogical alternative universe of medical billing.

When a medical provider sees you, she, of course, bills you. This is no different from what your plumber does. Each physician bill or "claim," as it is called in medicine, must have both an ICD code and a CPT code. The ICD code is your diagnosis when your saw your physician. ICD stands for International Statistical Classification of Diseases and Related Health Problems. It was created by the World Health Organization and now, is in its tenth revision. Therefore, it usually is written as ICD-10. This tenth revision of the code was begun in 1983 and completed in 1992. It is used throughout the world and was introduced in the United States on October 1, 2015. In theory, the use of the ICD-10 code makes sense. It can expedite medical insurance payment and it gathers medical statistics for studies. But like most things in American medicine, it is absurdly complex. For example, there are over 68,000 different codes in the system. This is in comparison to the ICD-9 system which had "only" 14,000. There are often multiple different codes for very similar diseases. This has led to more mistakes in medical coding and billing, which in turn leads to delays in payment and the adds to the expense for the whole system to fix those mistakes. The complexity of the system is demonstrated by the existence of some bizarre ICD-10 codes, which I have listed for your entertainment. (From Healthcare Dive, August 15, 2015).

Table 21. Some Bizarre Medical Billing Codes from ICD-10

V97.33XD	Sucked in jet engine, subsequent encounter
W51.XXA	Accidental striking against or bumped into by another person, sequala $32.10
V00.01XD	Pedestrian on foot injured in collision with roller-skater, subsequent encounter
Y93.D	Activities involved arts and handcrafts
Z99.89	Dependence on enabling machines and devises, not elsewhere classified
Y92.146	Swimming pool of prison as the place of occurrence of the exterior cause
S10.87XA	Other superficial bite of other specified part of neck, initial encounter
W61.62XD	Struck by duck, subsequent encounter

W55.41XA	Bitten by pig, initial encounter
Z63.1	Problems in relationships with in-laws
W220.2XD	Walked into lamppost, subsequent encounter
Y93.D:V91.07XD	Burn due to water-skis on fire, subsequent encounter
W55.29XA	Other contact with cow, subsequent encounter
W22.02XD: V95.43XS	Spacecraft collusion injuring occupant, sequela
W61.12XA	Struck by macaw, initial encounter
R46.1	Bizarre personal appearance

If you have ever wondered what your physician is doing when he is staring into his laptop instead of examining you after you have been sucked into a jet engine for a second time, he desperately is trying to find the right ICD-10 code for your diagnosis. But wait, we are not finished, for he also must find a CPT code for jet injury visit. CPT stands for Current Procedural Terminology and is a system developed by the American Medical Association. It is a huge database of the thousands of things that physicians do, professionally.

There are three major categories of CPT codes. Almost all things physicians do are found in Category I. Category II ones consist of extra notations sometimes added to a basic Category I code that shows extra steps the physician took during the evaluation. For example, the Category II code, 3006F, means a chest x-ray was reviewed and might be added to a code for treating pneumonia. Category III codes are for new and experimental therapies.

There are six sections of the Category I CPT code: evaluation and management, anesthesia, surgery, radiology, pathology and laboratory medicine, and general medicine. Each of the six sections is a nightmare of complexity of rules unto themselves, but the most commonly used one, evaluation and management (E/M) takes the prize. E/M is the billing code for what most physicians do most of the time. That is, find out what is wrong with a patient and come up with a plan to fix the problem. CPT E/M codes vary as to where the patient is located. There is a different code if the patient is in the hospital, office, emergency room, or nursing home. The code also varies is the patient is in the hospital as an admitted patient or under observation. The code varies if the patient is in a general hospital room or in intensive care. The code varies if the patient is seen as a consultation or not. A consultation simply means the patient was referred from another physician. The code varies if the patient is a new patient to the doctor or has been seen by her before. Of course, in our very surreal world of medical billing, if the patient has not been seen in three years by a physician, he is considered a "new" patient all over again.

For each of these possible locations of care, whether it is considered a new patient or not, and whether the visit is considered a consultation or not, there are five levels of care possible. For every increasing level of care a physician provides for a patient, she gets paid more. For there was more patient history taking, a more detailed physical examination and more complex medical decision making involved in the process. On paper, this seems like a very reasonable system.

Like many things in American medicine today, things are not what they appear to be and are never simple. The problem is that there is a required burdensome amount of documentation to prove you, the medical provider, have performed the level of care that you said that you did. You learn this when you sit in on too many "coding for dummies" classes, meant for us physicians. They drill into your cranium that if you did not document it on the patient's chart, it did not happen. Also, there is not uniformity for the same level of care. The requirements change, for example, if the patient is a new one or an existing one and if it is a consultation or not. Today's electronic medical records, instead of aiding the physician in the process of coding, add to this burden. The records demand a lot of input to create that paper trail for the documentation of the level of care. How much input? I once timed a true expert in CDT codes. She was a consultant, who specialized in reviewing medical charts and codes. This is what she did for a living, every day of her life. She could not code any medical record in under five minutes. Coding takes a lot of medical professionals' time.

We must add to that the *fear* factor. Many different types of bureaucrats audit medical records for the accuracy of the CPT codes. Which is ironic because they almost never audit charts for quality of care given to the patient. These auditors include ones from private medical insurance companies, Medicare and hospital networks. Improper coding is considered fraud and physicians can get huge fines and even go to prison if they are not performed properly.

What does all this coding work mean for medical care providers? It means practicing medicine, today in the United States, is like trying to land a Boeing 747 while at the same time texting five different people with a gun pointed at your head. Practicing medicine today is high pressure multi-tasking. If it appears that your physician is distracted while interacting with you in the office, emergency room or hospital, it is because he must think about coding and documentation for that coding at the same time he is thinking about your case, all the time he is worried that he will go to jail if he does it wrong. There are laws against texting and driving, as there should be. But why are there are no laws against distracted medicine while practicing coding?

Second, today's medical records primarily serve the need of coders and medical insurance companies. They are setup to please the billing bureaucrats. And you thought they were there to serve the needs of patients and their healthcare providers. One of the hardest, daily tasks in the practice of medicine is to review a patient's old medical records. That is because it is full of information that is only there to document for the insurance companies. It makes it hard to see the forest for the trees and find the pertinent information needed to treat the patient. The task is hard even when reviewing the records, the physician created herself or was created by her partner. It becomes doubly difficult if the records are from a different practice or hospital, where there usually is a completely different software system used for the records.

Pleasing the insurance gods with the documentation on the medical records leads to inaccuracies in "medical" side of things, too. In an effort to make sure things are documented correctly from a financial aspect, the physician often will quickly check off boxes on the electronic medical records or use what I call "copy and paste" documentation. When I was practicing gynecology, I cannot tell you how many times when I would review the medical records of a patient who had a hysterectomy in the past, find she had a "normal uterus" checked off on the electronic medical records of her last examination!

Third, valuable professional time is taken away from practice and education of real medicine. I cannot count the hundreds of hours I spent in classes, webinars, and one on one with billers reviewing my coding. All this was time I could have spent with patients or learning a new medical technique to truly help my patients. I recall one time I was sent to "coding summer school," because of my poor medical coding. I felt like such a dummy since I never failed a test in my life. But upon entering the class, I found my two classmates were the best physicians in our department, so I did not feel as bad about my need for this remedial training.

Fourth, physicians must hire billers and coders to submit their claims to medical insurance companies. Medical billing and coding have become so complicated, many, if not most physicians farm out the job to specialists to do the work for them. It is so complex that is cannot be done by the physicians' own staff anymore. That is why when you send in your payment to your physician, it typically goes to a bill collector in another state. This means that it costs money for physicians to collect their money. Of course, that extra cost is passed on to us, patients. And this becomes yet another reason American healthcare is so expensive compared with the rest of the world.

As bad as this complicated medical billing system, based on complex coding and documentation is, it is being slowly replaced by even more complicated systems. Several of them exist today. The oldest alternative model for fee-for-service is called capitation. With capitation, physicians are paid a fixed amount per month to take care of a patient. The payment is the same regardless of the number of times the patient is seen or even if the patient is not seen, at all. The payment typically varies based on demographics of the patient including factors like age and gender. Touted as a means to reduce costs, it in reality transfers the burden of insurance from the medical insurance company to the physician. The problem with such capitation systems is obvious. Patients who need a lot or complex care get short-changed. Because practitioners are not getting compensated, properly, they skimp on their care.

A second modern compensation system that modifies the fee-for-service model is the use of Relative Value Units (RVUs). Developed by Medicare, it assigns a number to each of the over nine thousand services and procedures that physicians do. The RVU is based on three components: the physician's work required to perform the service, the expenses of the procedure to the practice to do the service and the cost of malpractice insurance. The physician's work, in term, is based on the four subcomponents: the time it takes to perform the service, the technique skill and physical effort to perform the service, the amount of mental effort and judgment involved, and the stress arising from any potential complication to the patient from performing the service. For example, a typical office visit for an established patient has an RVU of 0.97 while the same level for a new patient has a value of 1.47. That means it supposedly takes 50% more time and effort to see a new patient to the practice rather than an established one. RVUs typically are used today to pay physicians who work for hospitals, networks or in large practices.

RVUs are all the rage in medical payments, today. I am not sure, why. They are just another complicated fee-for-service model with a three-letter name. RVUs do nothing to address the complexity of medical documentation for billing services. If anything, they encourage physicians to "pick and choose" what tasks they are going to perform. High value RVSs are being cherrypicked from low value ones. It also encourages what is wrong about the pace of medical care, today. They reward volume of care, not thoughtful medical practice.

Finally, there is Pay for Performance (P4P) model of compensation. This is a bonus system based on the quality of care, added to the traditional fee for service system. The medical insurance company evaluates the provider on four different metrics. First is called "process," that is, doing things make patients healthier, like handing out a prescription for a mammography for women over age 40 years. The second is "outcome," which is the actual achievement of that health goal. An example of this would be the percentage of women who received that prescription that had a mammography performed. The third is "patient satisfaction," which medicine's Open Table or Amazon Review equivalent. Surveys are taken as to how happy patients are in receiving their care from the practice. Wait times, staff helpfulness and communications are just a few of things measured. Now you know why you get so many phone calls, e-mails and snail mail about the quality of your medical service. They are just like the service department at your car dealership. Both are paid based on your perception of them. The final parameter is structural, an evaluation of the actual facilities including medical records.

On paper, P4P seems like a good idea. It rewards quality, not just quantity of medical care. In reality, it is much like those standardized tests that your children take in school to assess the quality of their education. Just like teachers "teach for the test," medical providers "work for the P4P bonus." Because only a narrow range of parameters can be and are measured, providers concentrate just on those goals, often ignoring other ones that are not.

Let me give you an example from my own experience from my obstetrician days. One P4P our old practice was measured and possibly rewarded for, was the percentage rate of our pregnant patients that were offered the flu vaccine. This "process" goal was an appropriate one. Such vaccinations reduce the incidence of influenza among pregnant women. This is a time when the disease can be more severe. The vaccine also can provide some passive immunity against influenza for the newborn after delivery. As the time for the goal neared, our groups' physicians would spend many hours checking to see if the flu vaccine offer was documented on every pregnant woman's medical record. Remember, the rules. It is not important that it was offered, it had to be documented, too! If it wasn't documented, we became like Captain Ahab, tracking down that patient to see if she had been offered the vaccine or not, so we could check that box on her medical record. I often wondered what other important medical activities we were neglecting while we were reenacting a scene from Moby Dick.

This longwinded review of how medical providers are paid demonstrates that paying for a parameter just does not work. Whether it is traditional fee for service with all their CDT codes, RVUs or P4P, it adds a needless complexity to the practice of medicine. It rewards high volume, cattle shoot practice, creates confusing and inaccurate medical records and adds to the cost of medicine. There must be a better way. Remember, there is the third way people are paid. Physicians and other medical providers should be paid for their *time*.

How would a time-based payment system function under

our proposed SPUN Insurance Plan? I am not proposing that physicians become hourly rate employees. Rather, when they are taking care of a patient, they are paid for the actual time they spend with them. Hear me out. First, procedures, like surgery, would be reimbursed like they are today. Each one would have a specific set fee attached to it. Whether it be removing a skin mole in the office or performing a heart transplant, there would be one fee assigned to the procedure for the total physician care in performing the procedure.

Second, there still would be diagnosis codes when a patient sees a health provider. These codes will serve several purposes. They will ensure that the fee submitted is in tune for the severity of the diagnosis. They will provide a "bookmark" in the medical records. They will make it easier to find this information in the future information, when a practitioner or patient is looking for it. Finally, these diagnosis codes will help for data mining from the complete collection of medical records. With a vast database of the entire country's medical records, future researchers will have a treasure trove of information about how to diagnosis and treat disease. But we need a much simpler and intuitive system than ICD-10. The diagnosis codes should serve the providers and patients, not the billers and the bureaucrats. Let us create a system of diagnosis codes that are far fewer in number and are based on how physicians think about disease.

Third, non-procedural medical billing will be strictly based on the provider's time. It would not matter if the patient is being seen in the office or in the hospital, is a new patient to the practitioner or an established one, if the patient is a consultation from another physician or not. For common sense tells us that one minute of physician time is just as valuable (or not valuable!) as every other. Let us make it "KISS" simple and pay a physician, at the same rate, regardless of what he was doing.

Fourth, the payment rate will be a per minute one. With modern computers, it is just as easy to measure small lengths of time as large ones, so let us be as precise as possible. Afterall, a lot of our money is at stake. Practitioners multitask. They will go from examining one patient, then answering a phone call from another and back to examining that first patient. Our system must capture these tiny aliquots of time that are spent on each patient.

Fifth, there will be a maximum time allowed to be billed. That time will be based on the diagnosis. For example, the maximum time allowed for the evaluation and treatment of a common cold will be less than for pneumonia. These maximum time allotments will be generous. We want to encourage physicians to slow down and take care of and listen to patients. In the long run, this will save the system money. For by spending more time with patients, physician trust is created. A good medical history, the key to most diagnoses, is elicited. There will be less need for testing, as physicians will be less inclined to shotgun it. And for the same reason, there will be fewer follow-up consultations for the same problem and referrals to other physicians.

Sixth, as we have noted, the physician also will collect a co-pay for most patient encounters. This would help strike a balance between carwash, assembly line medicine, where patients are rushed through as quickly as possible to generate more revenue and creating physicians who are government workers who milk the clock seeing as few patients a day as possible. There needs to be an incentive in the SPUN healthcare model to motivate the health providers to see a reasonable number of patients. The co-pay act as a bonus, in addition, to time paid, to prevent featherbedding.

Seventh, all time that the physician spends on a patient's case will count as time that would be reimbursed. That would work we, as patients, do not see that goes on behind the scenes. This includes reviewing old medical records, interpreting laboratory and radiology tests, talking with family members about the patient's care and phone calls with patients. Our American healthcare system reform must encourage out of office communication among health providers and patients. As things stand today, both sides have legitimate gripes and that is why the system is broken. Physicians complain that the extra time they spend on a patient's case outside of the actual encounter is not compensated. That is why they do not return your phone call promptly. No one likes working for free. Patients, on the other hand, complain that they cannot get hold of their providers in a timely manner. Remember this lack of physician-patient communication builds a Berlin Wall in the relationship. I believe paying for time spent on a patient's care outside of the office and hospital will be the Ronald Reagan in healthcare, tearing down that divisive wall.

Many practitioners-patient encounters need not be face to face. Too many patients today are brought into the doctor's office for very simple medical problems that could be handled by other means of communication. This wastes society's time, meaning it wastes all our time. We can start with the not so modern electronic communication, invented in 1876, the telephone. Five minutes of phone time can be just as valuable as five minutes of face to face time. Often patients come into a physician's office just to discuss a problem and no physical examination is performed. For example, they want to discuss how to lower their blood cholesterol level or about their insomnia. Certainly, these encounters can be handled over the phone.

A step up in technology would be for physicians and patients to communicate with video chatting. Skype and Facetime come to my mind. Thanks to modern smartphones, they could see, as well as talk to each other. Like the old saying goes, a picture is worth a thousand words. This could save many an office visit for a simple skin rash or a check of a surgical incision. Physicians could use this technology before referring a patient to another specialist. For example, while a patient is still in the office, a video chat with a specialist could be done right then and there. The specialist could render her opinion without having to physically see the patient. Obviously, this technology could not be used in most medical cases but think how efficient medical care could be even if it were used in just ten percent. That is 10% less time patients would have to spend taking off from work and sitting in crowded offices.

Eighth, other medical providers will be paid on their own unique per minute scale, based on their degree, training and ability. Much of today's medical care is provided by non-physicians who either supplement or replace that of doctors. This includes that provided by medical assistants, who gather information and take a preliminary history for the medical providers before the main encounter. Their time and talent should be compensated, separately, by the system. Encouraging the use of their talents frees up the scarcer resource of physician time. This is no different than in the legal field where the time a paralegal spends on your case is billed at a separate, lower rate from the actual lawyer handling you care. Today, medical assistants are overworked. That is why they usually seems rushed when they bring you back for your office visit. That is because their services are not compensated for today with our present medical insurance payment system. By paying for their services, separately, their bosses (physicians) then would be encouraging them to spend more time with you and that encounter will be more valuable.

Registered nurses perform valuable triage tasks in physician practices. Armed with just a phone and a patient's medical records, they usually are the first line of help in office medical care. They are the first medical voice, patients hear when they are ill. When fully and properly utilized, they provide valuable medical care, deciding on an initial plan of action for the ill patient. They decide if, when, where and how soon, ill patients are seen. During my years of obstetric and gynecologic practice, I was lucky enough to work with one of the finest phone nurses, Cindy Butterworth. With her training, self-education, compassion, unmatched experience, tireless work ethic and sense of humor, she was one of the best practitioners of medicine I ever met, even though she was "just a nurse." Even when I had been in practice for decades, I would seek out her advice when I had a difficult case, because I knew she would have the answer. The best medical care does not necessarily have an M.D. after its name. Our SPUN medical care system, by compensating registered nurses for their time and talent and our professional license system, by allowing them to do more of what they can do, should encourage the creation of more Cindy Butterworths. We all would be healthier because of it and spend less money doing so.

Mid-level providers are a present-day example of wisely using non-physician resources. Nurse practitioners, physician assistants and nurse midwives are called "physician extenders." On any given day, when I practiced medicine, approximately 80% of my tasks could be handled by these near physicians. Mid-level providers are a true "win-win" for a healthcare system. They are far less expensive to pay for their services that physicians usually do and they free up scarce physician time, for things they cannot do. Let us give these mid-level providers even more professional freedom. Let us encourage more of them to enter the field so we can make even more use of them in medicine.

Finally, there is a wide range of other health providers, whose professional services will be covered under our SPUN Healthcare Plan. Think dentists, podiatrists, optometrists, behavioral health specialists, physical and occupation therapists, just to name a few. Let us simplify the medical billing for all of them. Let us pay them for their time at an appropriate rate under the same system that we will pay physicians.

You may ask how we are going to figure out that professional time to do the medical billing. That brings us to the ninth tenet of our billing system. Professional time will be tracked by the SPUN Healthcare Plan electronic medical records (EMR). It would be a simple task for all involved. Afterall, my iPhone tells me each day how many minutes and seconds I spend on Facebook. Let our medical record system automatically time when a certain patient's medical record is being accessed by that provider. The EMR would keep track of all the practitioner's patients' encounters, at the end of a day create a time report to send to SPUN for billing. Instead of medical records being a beast to be tamed in medical billing, working against the practitioner, let it be a beast of burden (Sorry Mick.) simplifying the billing process.

You may say I am too pie in the sky. You may ask for an example of such a billing system that I am proposing that exists today. There is such a professional billing model that pays for all time and effort spent on a case. It is the way most lawyers bill for their work. If it works for them and in other professions like consulting, it should work in medicine, too.

This time-based system would have many benefits beyond just simplifying medical billing. We finally would get the time and consideration from our medical providers that we deserve as patients. Remember our example of paying your children by the hour to rake leaves. Paying by time encourages slow, deliberate work. Medicine is not like assembling toys in a Third World sweat factory. It is based on a unique relationship that requires dedicated time to build. Freed of the need to please the insurance billers and coders, the encounter would not be a multitasked one. Multitasking is fine for computers but not humans. We work better performing one task at a time. Medicine must slow down. Finally, just maybe you would learn the color of your physician's eyes or have a real conversation with your medical assistant.

Medical records would return to their original task, medical records. They would not exist to be an insurance validation service. Future medical records will be an efficient vault of a patient's health and disease history that is an easily assessable archive for the patient and her health providers.

Billing costs will plummet. Our three-way chess game played among patient, provider and insurance company will disappear. Providers will not need a huge billing staff to create claims. Our SPUN Health Insurance plan employees will not need an army of clerks to process the claims and answer telephone calls from confused and frustrated patients.

When it was time to adjust how much the SPUN plan would pay, this would be a simple task. All the system would have to do is change the per minute payment amount. Just one number would have to be recalculated.

Our system could be used to encourage practitioners to practice in underserved areas or in underserved professions. Today's payers, including medical insurance companies and Medicare, pay more to practitioners who practice in high expense areas, like large cities and suburban areas. The purpose is to compensate them for the higher cost of living in these areas. This is backward thinking. Today, large cities and suburbs have an adequate or even an oversupply of physicians. These parts of our country do not need subsidies for attracting medical talent. Our SPUN Insurance Plan would pay every practitioner in the country at the same rate, regardless of where they practice. This will encourage practitioners to seek out the lower cost of practicing medicine, rural areas of the country that are underserved.

If our system still identifies parts of our country that have too few providers, flat-rate, yearly bonuses will be offered to attract more physicians. These bonuses will continue as long as the practitioner practiced in an underserved area. It will be an easy task to identify these parts of the country. Having a single insurance provider, one database of all national health services will make this analysis a snap.

This high need area, bonus system will replace our present student loan forgiveness programs. Loan forgiveness programs were created as a response to the huge student debt, future physicians accumulate. You think you have huge college loans to repay? Think again. Today, the typical medical student graduate has $189,000 in debt from their student loans (2017 data from the Association of American Medical Colleges). Physicians, after finishing their residencies for their specialty training, often will sign up for several years with the one of the branches of the armed forces, the Indian Health Services, or another national or state sponsored programs. In turn for working in such programs for a fixed amount of time, part or all their medical school student loans are forgiven. But there is a problem with such loan forgiveness programs as they are today. Most of these newly minted physicians will leave the underserved program after they do their time and their debt forgiven. Turnstile medical care results. This affects the continuity of care, critical in underserved, impoverished areas. Remember medical care is about building and *maintaining* relationships.

Today's high student debts attract physicians into high income, specialty areas. You cannot blame them. They are not just being mercenary; they must pay off their debt somehow. Therefore, society winds up with more plastic surgeons than it needs. But what the United States really needs is more primary care physicians (family medicine physicians, internists, pediatricians) and psychiatrists. These, traditionally, are lower salaried fields of medicine.

Also, many bright, altruistic and motivated young people are deterred from even seeking a medical education in the first place, fearing the huge medical debt load in their futures. Why become a physician when the cost of education to be an investment banker is so much less? The solution again is simple and commonsense. The rest of the high-income world subsidizes the cost of physician education. We should, too, down at least to a reasonable tuition rate.

This would just be the first step in reducing our national physician shortage. We must retain the services of the physicians that society already has trained for as long as we can. Physician burnout is a real problem, at a crisis point in the United States. Unfortunately, it is one not talked about very much. Why? As physicians, we are told to "just suck it up or there is the door!" There is not much empathy for a group that is supposed to be so empathetic. Therefore, the burnout problem does not get the attention it deserves. How bad is the problem? A Medscape study looked at physician burnout rates in 27 different medical specialties for 2017. Physicians were asked to rate their degree of burnout on a one to seven scale. One on the scale means it does not interfere at all with the physician's professional life while seven means the physician is thinking of quitting the field, entirely. The results of the Medscape study revealed that all, but one specialty field, scored an average score of four or higher. The highest burnout fields are emergency medicine, obstetrics and gynecology, family medicine and internal medicine. The top four causes of burnout are: too many bureaucratic tasks, too many hours of work, the feeling of just being a cog in the wheel and the computerization of medical practice.

Notice what is *not* on the list of causes of physician burnout. It is not the malpractice crisis or fear of lawsuits. It is not demanding patients or 4 am telephone calls. It is not the stress of always being the umpire in the bottom of the ninth inning at the seventh game of the World Series; making the tough calls that physicians must make. Physicians want to be physicians. They want to take care of patients.

Notice the common theme of physician's complaints on our list. They do not like doing things that takes them from direct patient care. A recent time and motion study conducted by the

AMA and the Dartmouth-Hitchcock Health Care System found that only 27% of physician's work time is spent on direct clinical care. American physicians, today, are cooks who are rarely in the kitchen, baseball players who are always sitting on the bench, and actors who are building the sets for the stage. Imagine a world where that number is 75%. A world where physicians spend three-quarters of their time taking care of patients instead of just one-quarter as it is today. In theory, we would need only half as many physicians and we still would get 50% more time with those we have! And as a bonus, all physicians would be happier and not want to go work at the local Home Depot. (Do not laugh. I know a physician who did just that.)

The second step in reducing our national physician shortage is to shift more clinical and non-clinical tasks to other medical professionals. Did you ever have a new garbage disposal put in your house? A plumber comes to do the actual installation, but an electrician must make a separate visit to hook up the two simple electric wires to complete the job. It is not that the plumber cannot do the simple wiring, it is just their "trade rules" will not allow it. That is nothing compared to what exists in American medicine today. There are hundreds of different types of medical professionals that practice today. Specialization can be a good thing as the practitioner can get really good at the very intricate tasks and services that medicine demands. However, overspecialization also creates rigid boundaries where professionals are not permitted or are afraid to do anything that is "not in their job description." Today, rigid hospital and practice rules and policies, state licensure practices and medico-legal concerns all get in the way of commonsense.

Let me give a few examples. Let us start with my practicing specialty of obstetrics. On many labor and delivery floors, obstetric nurses are not permitted to check a laboring woman's cervical dilatation. As any woman who ever had a baby will tell you, how far the cervix is open is a critical obstetric measurement. Often, cervical dilatation must be assessed quickly. Obstetric nurses are with the patient in labor almost continually. Those professionals, obstetricians, obstetric residents and midwives, that can perform the check of the cervix usually are not readily assessable, delaying patient care, sometimes resulting in negative outcomes. Plus, obstetric nurses are permitted to make much more difficult assessments in a woman's labor management, like interpreting the fetal electronic heartrate tracing. Finally, assessing a cervix of a laboring patient is not rocket science; it is an easily learned skill. Common sense says it should not be limited to physicians.

Here is another example from obstetrics. In 1989, the third year I was in obstetric practice, a landmark article was published by the National Institute of Health in Bethesda, Maryland concerning prenatal care (Caring for our future: The content of prenatal care. A report of the public health expert panel on the content of prenatal care.) The article combined the opinions of dozens of experts with the review of thousands of scholarly articles to study everything that was ever published about care of pregnant women before labor and delivery. Not surprisingly, it emphasized the importance and cost-effectiveness of such care. What *was* surprising was that the report suggested radical changes in how prenatal care is given in the United States. One of the report's conclusions was that most of prenatal care could be and should be given by non-physicians. That included registered nurses, nurse practitioners, physician assistants, nurse midwives and nutritionists. That is because the education of pregnant patients is such a critical component of prenatal care. Such education takes time, a lot of it. The best professionals to provide such time would be non-physicians, who have more time to give such education. Also, shifting who is giving prenatal care would save the entire healthcare system money. Although during my career I saw some baby steps (pun intended) toward this goal, by the time I retired from obstetrics in 2016, the vast majority of prenatal care still was being performed by obstetricians. Once again, common sense was ignored.

Moving on to an example from the behavioral health field. Today, in the United States, there are two major groups of mental health specialists. There are psychiatrists and non-psychiatrists. Psychiatrists are physicians with specialty training in the field which they complete after medical school. They prescribe medications but often do not counseling. Psychiatric nurse practitioners or physician assistants may supplement their duties and also can prescribe medications. The second "non-physician" group includes clinical psychologists with a doctoral degree (PhD.) in psychology, clinical social workers, counselors with a master's degree in social work who usually works in a hospital setting, licensed professional counselors, mental health counselors and nurse psychotherapists, all with master's degrees in their fields. In general, this second group of therapists are not allowed to prescribe medications. This split in duties right down the middle of the behavioral health field creates a huge inefficiency. Not surprisingly, patients with mental health disorders usually need both counseling and medications. But today, they cannot get it by one stop shopping. This leads to these patients not getting the healthcare they need and when they do, it is a lot more expensive than it need be.

The solution is obvious. We should allow non-psychiatrists to prescribe psychiatric medications. Of course, there would be limitations and regulations, but common sense should prevail. There has been a push in the United States to permit this to happen, called the prescriptive authority for psychologist movement. The arguments for such prescribing include the fact that other non-physicians can prescribe medications, including dentists, pharmacists, podiatrists, optometrists, nurse practitioners and physician assistants. Psychologists easily could be trained in the necessary basic science of pharmacology. Such prescribing would ease the nationwide and in particular, rural shortage of psychiatrists. There would no longer need to be the difficult coordination of care between psychiatrist and non-psychiatrist. But best of all, it would ease the task of obtaining healthcare for those who have had it the worst, those with mental health disease, by making one visit out of two.

When you go to the dentist for your twice a year checkup, most of the visit is performed by the dental hygienist. That including the cleaning, oral health screening, education and x-rays. Your dentist comes in at the very end for your final dental examination and to consult with you if you have any problems. Most of the dentist's day is spent taking care of dental problems: filling cavities, making crowns and pulling teeth.

Let us contrast that with your typical visit to your primary care provider. When you go to your family doctor or internist's practice for a routine checkup, you usually see your physician. But if you have an acute medical problem, you are seen by the practice's physician assistant or nurse practitioner. This is because the mid-level providers have more time in their schedules and it is easier to fit your problem into their schedules. This is backward medicine. We need a dental model of medical care to best utilize the talents and education of our physicians and midlevel providers. It makes much more sense to see the midlevel provider for your routine checkup. That way, they can spend more time with you, especially for the needed component of health education. And you should see a physician when you have a medical problem because they have more professional resources and training to help you with that problem. Again, it is just common sense.

So far, we have been just talking about easing the burden of clinical tasks for the physician. What can be done to ease physicians and other health professionals of *non*-clinical tasks? We already have documented that physicians spend three-quarters of their work time on non-clinical tasks. We have compared this to having LeBron James sell basketball tickets in the booth before playing the game. (One article actually made that comparison. Forbes September 7, 2016, Doctors wasting over two-thirds of their time doing paperwork.) Physician time is too scarce a commodity and too expensive to use on such non-clinical tasks. Society should not be paying doctors $200 to $400 an hour to fill out school physical forms. Remember, every minute a physician spends on paperwork is a minute not spend on patient care. The solution is simple and twofold. Reduce the total amount of medical paperwork that exists and offload much of the rest to non-physicians.

You are asking what can be done to reduce the volume of non-clinical physician work. My answer: combine and simplify. Today, physicians must please many masters as they go about their work: their employers, health insurance companies, local, state and federal governments, the hospitals where they practice, and the professional organizations run by their profession and their specialties. Each has their own set of rules, that often overlap and conflict with one another. Today, it a burdensome challenge for health professionals figure out all the rules and keep in compliance with them.

Let me start by giving you one personal example. All actively practicing physicians are required to take a certain number of hours of continuing medical education (CME). Of course, this makes sense. You want your doctors to stay up to date with the ever-changing practice of medicine. However, the CME requirements for number of hours and type of education are not uniform. The state of Pennsylvania, where I practiced, Abington Jefferson, the hospital network where I worked, the American Medical Association, the general physician national organization, and the American College of Obstetrics and Gynecology, the specialty national organization, each have their own CME rules and requirements. Often, for the same education activity, one organization would classify the number of hours toward the goal, differently from another. Back when I was practicing medicine, every time I did a continuing education activity, I entered the data into four different spreadsheets to keep track of it for my four different masters. And of course, these CME requirements changed over time.

The license to practice medicine is granted by the individual states. However, the ability to write prescriptions for controlled medications, a critical activity required of all physicians is separate. It is maintained by the Drug Enforcement Agency (DEA) and is a federal one. That means every physician must maintain and renew two licenses. It also means that if a physician wishes to move her practice out of state, she must apply for a new license in that state. And you guessed it, the requirements for a medical license differ from state to state.

Today, to be paid by the medical insurance companies, they must qualify you as a provider into their plans. You guessed it, again. There is a separate application for each medical insurance plan and these, too, must be renewed, periodically.

Having one universal set of professional requirements, established by the SPUN Insurance Program, will go a long way to create more precious physician clinical time. This is an example of a time that it would be better to tear down the house and build a new one, rather than try to make repairs to our present one. Let us start over from the foundations with all professional requirements. First, let us eliminate all the complex, multiple and conflicting requirements for medical professionals of the local, state and federal governments, hospitals and health networks, health insurance plans, medical and professional organizations. We will replace them with one set of simple, national, uniform requirements maintained by SPUN.

In addition to eliminating many non-clinical tasks, physicians should be able to offload more of it, too. Physicians are the only professionals who do not have real administrative assistants. True, we are aided by office managers, billing clerks, receptionists, office nurses and medical assistants. However, none of this group eases our non-clinical duties like an administrative assistant would do for an accountant or lawyer. Typically, a lot of physician time is spent on mundane tasks. Hours of physician time was spent in my old practice creating on call and office schedules for physicians. Precious time was spent on the telephone, on hold, tracking down lost patient laboratory and pathology reports. The end of every day in the office was met with a pile of disability and similar forms that needed to be completed (and were done so, usually poorly). In addition to completing complex and lengthy medical records, physicians compose letters to consultants and referring physicians, often typing and mailing the letters, themselves. Physicians spend time scheduling tests and procedures for patients. Sometimes, I would spend more time trying to coordinate the timing of a cesarean section than it took to actually perform the surgery. Physicians make their own phone calls and often are on hold on the telephone waiting to speak to other physicians doing similar tasks. Physicians often are reluctant to call other physicians because they know how busy they must be with administrative tasks and do not want to burden them more. Many physicians still own their own practices or if they work for a hospital or network, still need to run their practices. That means, a lot of their time is spent on human resource matters like the hiring and evaluation of employees, office finances and the day to day running of their practices.

This terrible situation is more than just a waste of precious physician clinical time. For physicians typically are only good at being physicians and not much else. That is why many physician practices are chaotically run. All physician practices, from the smallest rural solo practitioner to the largest national physician network, should take a long hard look at how their practices are organized and how personnel are utilized. Practices, today, have a clinical staff and a non-clinical staff. An office manager, at the top of the organization's chart, does a lot of the day to day running of the practice. The clinical staff consists of the physicians, mid-level providers (physician assistants, midwives and nurse practitioners), nurses and medical assistants. The non-clinical staff consists of a billing staff and receptionists. The non-clinical staff usually have no formal training and typically learn as they go. They are overworked, low paid and have a high turnover rate.

A new role of medical administrative assistant would replace most of the duties of today's not-clinical staff. Since insurance billing will be much easier under SPUN, they can ease the non-clinical burdens of practicing physicians. Such an assistant would have formal training as a two-year program at a high school tech school or as an associate degree at a community college. Medical administrative assistants (MMAs) would learn the complex world of medical practices. Their education would include electronic scheduling, medical records and medical insurance. (Of course, medical insurance will be much easier to learn with SPUN than it is today!) At work, MMAs would shadow the practicing doctor. In addition to typical receptionist's duties, they would schedule tests for patients, compose and send out referral letters, make phone calls and organize the physician's work day. All with the goal of letting the physician be a physician. With more responsibilities and more training would come better pay and benefits for MMAs. But it would be cost-effective as physicians would have more time with patients.

You may object that the proposed SPUN Healthcare System has no incentives for quality of care in its compensation program for physicians and other providers. But, yes, dear reader, it does. By giving the provider more time to practice medicine and rewarding the practitioner who spends more time with patients, this will stimulate better quality medical care. This is more important and more likely to improve healthcare than setting up a few arbitrary metrics that physicians now are judged upon and they can skirt around.

That does not mean the quality of provider care is not going to be evaluated by SPUN. Because there will be just one insurance provider in the United States and one set of uniform medical records, it will be easy to obtain a treasure trove of quality data on physicians and other healthcare providers. Some would be for all practitioners, regardless of specialty and include things like length of time to obtain an appointment, office wait time, average time spent with patient, average time to return phone calls and practitioner's patient volume, just to name a few. Other metrics would be specific to the specialty. For example, as an obstetrician-gynecologist, I would be rated on number of deliveries performed per year, cesarean section rate, episiotomy rate, obstetric complication rate, hysterectomy rate, just to name a few.

This information would be public, not unlike similar data that is available on line when we search for a hotel room at Expedia, a restaurant at Open Table or a book at Amazon. It would serve two major purposes. First, it would be an informational source for patients. Today, patients typically pick their doctors the same way they did one hundred years, ago. That is, by word of mouth. They get recommendations from family and friends or from another medical practitioner. Although, there are several websites where patients can go to rate their physicians, these sites do not provide much information about the quality of care. All physicians have unique medical skills and interests. Patients should be able to seek out these skills to fit their specific needs. For example, if a woman needs a hysterectomy, she should be able to easily find a gynecologist who has performed a lot of this type of surgery with a low complication rate. Second, this quality information would be used to make sure a practitioner meets a minimum standard to practice. Presently, physicians and other practitioners must go through several different hoops to stay in practice. That includes the ability to practice at their hospital (called hospital privileges), state licensure requirements, and requirements for the various medical insurance companies that they have agreed to participate in their plans. The professional credentialing process is redundant and arbitrary. More importantly, it is not very useful to weeding out the bad apples in the field. Having one and only one process, based on a practitioner's total volume of work, will be a much fairer and simpler system and one that would assure the public the physicians they see are competent to practice medicine. More of this topic, later in this book.

We have finished our discussion on how medical practitioners will be compensated in the future, under our SUPN Healthcare System. Let us turn our attention to how hospitals should be paid for their services. Hospital fees are separate from physician fees. For example, if you have surgery performed in a hospital, there are two fees: one for the surgeon and one for the hospital. How do hospital bills work, today? Today, hospitals bill patients like hotels bill their guests that stay with them. There is a daily rate for the length of the stay and additional fees for the extras. Instead of a tab from the mini-bar or for Wi-Fi, hospitals bill for such services as laboratory tests, x-rays, medications, intravenous fluids, medical supplies, and operating room time. These additional hospital fees are listed on what is called the chargemaster or charge description master (CDM). Yes, there is yet another three letter anacronym we must learn. Each hospital maintains its own CDM and it usually contains 20,000 to 50,000 different costs. CDMs are yet another level of unneeded complexity in our healthcare system/ Hospital employees spend a significant portion of their professional time scanning barcodes and clicking computer keyboards when they are taking care of patients to make sure every item on that list is captured for billing.

As we have seen, these daily rates and CDM fees are just a retail price. Very few patients ever will pay them. That is why you often hear of the $25 bill for a single Tylenol tablet from a hospital. Medical insurance companies negotiate what they pay with the hospitals, and it is just a fraction of the CDM fees. Of course, each insurance company that a hospital deals with will pay a different amount for the same charge. It is just like when you buy a new car. Three different customers will pay three different prices for the exact model automobile.

Medicare, a significant revenue source for hospitals, works differently (of course) from the private insurances when it comes to hospital billing and payment. The government pays based on something called the Inpatient Prospective Payment System. This system first assigns every hospital bill a diagnosis related group (DRG). This is the primary diagnosis for the hospitalized patient from one of 700 different ones. The more serious the DRG, the higher the Medicare payment. For example, the DRG for a myocardial infarction is going generate a higher payment than for gallstones. This base payment then is adjusted for each individual hospital, based on the hospital's expenses, whether the hospital is a teaching one or not, or if the hospital has a high rate of low-income patients. The payment may be adjusted for various hospital performance criteria, too.

There is a major problem with this Medicare and Medicaid hospital payment system as it exists today. Although they operate under a system similar to our proposed plan, they do not even cover the hospital's costs for treating the patient, let alone allow the hospital to generate a profit. According to the American Hospital Association Annual Survey of United States Hospitals for 2015, Medicare reimbursement was $41.6 billion less than the costs for the hospital to treat the patients. That means Medicare and Medicaid payments do not cover the expenses for personnel pay and benefits, hospital equipment and running costs. Doing a bit of arithmetic, we find Medicare only pays 88 cents for every dollar spent by the hospital to take care of a Medicare patient. And according to the Congressional Budget Office, this gap is going to grow worse in the future.

Remember hospitals also lose money taking care of patients who do not have medical insurance or are underinsured and have large out of pocket costs and do not pay their bills. That means hospitals, to stay in business, must make up the loss on Medicare, Medicaid and uninsured patients by overcharging those with private insurance. That is the problem when a country has three different ways of paying hospital bills. The uninsured are billed retail, but rarely are able to pay their bills. Those on governmental plans are paid under a fairly simple system based on their diagnosis, but it does not cover the hospital's costs. The insured are billed based on a complex system that captures every expense they incur in the hospital, but pay at a reduced cost, but not that reduced since it must cover the loss generated by the other two groups. Are you confused by it all? Of course.

The problems that modern American hospitals face go beyond how they are paid. For they are eighteenth century structured institutions trying to survive in a twenty-first century world. To understand these problems, we must review a brief history of hospitals and how they evolved in the United States to where they are today. The early American colonies took a cue from Europe where there was a Christian charity tradition. The Church, throughout its history, would reach out to help feed and clothe the poor, care for widows and children, and offer hospitality to strangers. This charity tradition also included taking care of the sick. That is why so many hospitals today have an association with various Christian and other religious groups. The colonies had almshouses whose primary mission was custodial care for the poor but included care for the sick among them. Benjamin Franklin, when he was not busy being a printer, postmaster, starting the American Revolution and flying a kite, was founding the first true hospital in the United States. This was Pennsylvania Hospital, established in 1751, and still an institution in Philadelphia, today.

For the next century and a half in the United States,

hospitals remained charitable institutions. Only the poor received care, there. The rest of society received medical care at home, given by their families and supervised by visiting physicians. (This was the origin of the old-fashioned doctor house call.) There was no professional nursing staff or care. Birth and death occurred at home. Even surgery was performed in the home. Hospitals gained a reputation as places poor people went to die. I still remember this attitude toward hospitals in the views of my grandparents who justifiably had a morbid fear of them.

Slowly, three major groups of hospitals developed There were privately-supported voluntary hospitals, usually supported by Protestant religious sects. They were managed by trustees and funded by donations to them. Second, there were Catholic hospitals, entirely run and staffed by brothers and sisters of the church. They were supported by fundraising. Finally, there were public hospitals that were supported by local taxes. The first two were the origin of today's non-profit hospitals and the last, the origin of today's urban, public hospitals. Regardless of whether they were non-profit or public, their work was charity work. Patients rarely paid for hospital services.

The time from the start of the twentieth century through World War II saw a dramatic change in the mission of American hospitals. They evolved into places where sick people of all economic classes could get better instead of just die. Therefore, the demand for their services exploded. For example, the number of hospital beds in the country increased six times faster than the growth of the population in the years between 1909 and 1932. The reason for the changes in the mission of hospitals was the advance in medical technology. Nursing, for example, became a skilled profession with a defined training curriculum. There were the new medical advances of diagnostic x-rays and laboratory testing. Sterile technique and modern anesthesia meant surgery now was far safer in the hospital than in the home.

The advent of Blue Cross medical insurance plans during

this same era meant that hospitals were now being paid for their services and becoming less pure charitable institutions. The creation of Medicare and Medicaid during the 1960s meant the government was now involved, both as a payee and a regulator. It also meant that hospitals functioned more like businesses and less like philanthropic organizations. Not surprisingly, many became true businesses. That is to say, they were for profit companies, following the money.

You may ask what is the difference between non-profit and for-profit hospitals? On the surface, not much. Both have emergency rooms, operating suites and lousy hospital food. Both offer the same amount of charity care. Both deliver the same quality of service. Both have chief executive officers that make a lot of money, unlike what is seen with other non-health care non-profit organizations. For example, the head of the Stanford University Hospital System, Amir Dan Rubin, earned $3.1 million in 2012. This is more the president of the entire university, John Hennessy, made in 2016, which was a mere $1.2 million.

What is different between non-profit and for-profit hospitals is what you do not see behind the façade. It happens in the accounting departments. For for-profit institutions, well, profit is important. (I bet you can't say that last sentence five times fast.) Like all businesses, whether they be Apple making iPhones or your local bakery making donuts, they focus on this bottom line. Profit, from Accounting 101, is the difference between income that you make from your business and expenses that you incur running your business. For-profit hospitals have a laser focus on increasing income and reducing expenses. For example, compared to non-profit health systems, they are more likely to offer such medical services as open-heart surgery, a big money maker and less likely to offer substance abuse treatment, an unprofitable one. For-profit hospitals respond to these income and expense incentives more quickly than non-profits. For example, when home healthcare became a big moneymaker, for-profits were three times as likely to offer such services than non-profits. And when home healthcare became less lucrative, they were much more likely to drop it.

That extends to even whether to remain open, at all. For-profit institutions are more likely to close if they cannot meet expenses. This is because they answer to a board of directors and shareholders whose interest is profit, not like non-profit institutions, whose board of directors are members of the community, whose focus is medical service to the area.

The finances of for-profit and profit hospitals are different. One obvious difference is that for-profit hospitals pay corporate and property taxes. They also have more financial resources available to them when they need to raise money. For example, they can sell shares of stock while non-profits do not have stockholders.

Whether non-profit or for-profit, American hospitals faced major financial challenges, starting during the 1980s. The cash cow of private medical insurance companies and governmental funding of Medicare and Medicaid began giving less and less milk. Cost containment became the buzz word. Services were shifted as much as possible to the less expensive out of hospital or outpatient realm. Major restructuring occurred in the healthcare industry. Small hospitals could no longer compete and closed. Larger ones merged or bought each other out. Big fish hospitals swallowed smaller fish ones, only themselves to be swallowed by even bigger fish ones. This phenomenon still is happening today. For example, in the Philadelphia area, where I live and used to practice, the Jefferson Health System has emerged as a huge hospital network. Jefferson merged with Abington Health, just a few years after Abington acquired the even smaller community hospitals of Warminster Hospital and North Penn Hospital.

Ironically, it was at this time that the Certificate of Need

(CON) requirement for hospitals mostly was removed. To prevent excess medical care capacity in the form of hospital beds and expensive equipment, states enacted laws, called CON, that required hospitals prove their servicing communities needed the extra facilities. It became a national law, in 1974, called the National Health Planning and Resource Development Act. However, the law was repealed in 1987, taking the teeth out of the state laws. This led to hospitals adding excess capacity they did not need, at a time that demand for their services was falling.

Hospitals started to compete with one another for patients. They advertised their services, like retailers and banks, seemingly everywhere. One could not miss their ads, on line, on billboards and on the air. Hospitals purchased physician practices by the scores to both capture more patients and protect their patient base. They emphasized their non-medical strengths. It is not a coincidence that is when private patient rooms became common and huge hospital lobbies with marble fountains made their appearance.

Hospitals hired consultants to improve their bottom lines. That included experts both inside and outside of their four walls. A nurse manager's job traditionally was to run the nursing care in the various parts of the hospital, whether it be the delivery room, operating room, general medical and surgical floor or operating room. Now they were called upon to be bean counters, too, asked to look for ways to cut material and personnel costs for their departments. Physicians with MBA degrees were hired to run large out-patient networks that employed hundreds of doctors and other practitioners and had to figure ways of making them profitable. The Chief of Staff used to be the "head physician" in the hospital, charged with administrating clinical duties. That position changed to more of an economic one, figuring out what clinical areas made the hospital money and which ones did not.

High paid consultants from outside the hospital became

unseen but critical part of the organization. They made determinations about what parts of the hospital made money and what parts did not and therefore, what parts stayed opened and what parts closed. They made strategic pricing decisions, determining what to charge and how they could push the private and governmental insurance payers to pay more. They typically took a percentage cut of each price increase they created for the hospital.

That brings our tale of American hospitals to the present day. The demand for hospital services, especially in-patient services, still is going down. The total number of in-patient hospital days in the United States has dropped from 179,000,000 to 170,000,000 from the year 2008 to 2012. The total number of in-patient admissions dropped from 35,500,000 to 34,200,000 during this same period. Hospital bed occupancy rates have dropped from 77% in 1980 to 60% in 2013. All these statistics mean that there is an overcapacity of hospital services in our country. Why, you are asking? It is because more and more of modern medicine is performed out of the hospital, so-called "out-patient". For example, when my mother had her gallbladder removed in 1974, she spent 6 days in the hospital after a traditional open surgery. When I had my gallbladder removed in 2013, it was performed with me being an outpatient using laparoscopic, minimally invasive surgery.

Despite declining demand for their services, the human resources needed to run today's hospitals are increasing. For example, in 2008, there were 3,875,073 full-time hospital employees while in 2012, the number was 4,068,209. While in all other modern services and manufacturing industries, today's American worker grows more efficient, the modern American healthcare worker becomes less efficient in doing his job, each year. What does efficiency mean? If it is takes 100 hours to make the same car that used to take 200 hours, we would say efficiency of making a car has improved 50%. Think how barcode scanners improved the efficiency of the grocery store clerk and make it faster for you to check out and pay your grocery bill. In a million ways, small and big, techniques and technologies make our work more productive for the same amount of effort. That efficiency can be measured. It is a positive 1.8% per year in the United States and has been at approximately that rate for the past two decades. Turning back to healthcare. Not only is the efficiency rate less than 1.8% per year for American healthcare workers, it is actually a negative number. According to Robert Kocher of the Brookings Institute and Nikhil Sahni of Harvard University, it is a negative 0.6% a year.

That means, each year, it requires more people time to do the same medical task. Or put another way, each healthcare provider accomplished less each year, though she is working the same number of hours. Thanks to the power of compounding, that 0.6% loss in efficiency adds up to a significant number over time. Let me give you a personal example. As an obstetrician, I deliver babies. Let us say, my first year in private practice, 1986, I delivered 200 babies. Therefore, my last year in practice, 2016, I should have delivered only 162 babies for the same effort. That is why we see the paradox of the number of healthcare workers in hospitals increasing, and the output in terms of patient days in the hospital declining.

Let us sum up of the problems of American hospitals, today. They have excessive capacity. Their costs are increased because of declining efficiency. Finally, reimbursement rates are declining and highly variable based on payer. How will our SPUN Healthcare Plan pays hospitals should address these problems.

First, because SPUN will be a universal plan, all hospital bills will be paid at the same rate and there will be no non-payers. Hospitals will no longer have to have the loss leader of Medicare, Medicaid and charity cases that need higher reimbursement coverage by private insurers. One payer means the hospitals will not need a huge bureaucracy to submit claims and collect payments from multiple insurers, governmental agencies and patients. Administrative costs, a major contributor to the declining efficiencies of the American healthcare work, should plummet.

Second, hospitals will only have to answer to one set of master regulations, again our SPUN system. Today, hospitals, like we saw for physicians, have a bewildering array of local, state, federal governmental departments and regulations to address. They also must address accreditation and certification issues from private, non-profit organizations such as the Joint Commission. They must meet the different qualifications of dozens of private insurers. On the surface, it makes sense to ensure that hospitals are safe places. But with so many regulatory demands, often conflicting and reductant, hospitals are forced to concentrate more on meeting these demands than to cure patients. It is no different that the elementary student who is taught to pass the state-required standardized tests instead of just learn how to read, write and do math. Like for physicians, having one set of standards for hospitals to follow for accreditation, certification and reimbursement just is common sense. We will talk more about this simplification of our medical regulatory system in more detail, later in this book.

Third, it is time to end the concept of non-profit hospitals. Earlier in this book, when I proposed a national, single payer with universal coverage for the country, you probably thought I was a pink-o, socialist Communist. Now, you must think I am a right-wing, greedy, laisse-faire capitalist. But hear me out for what I really am is a practicalist with a touch of cynicism mixed in. With the SPUN Healthcare Plan paying for virtually all services, the charity aspect of hospitals will no longer be needed. We do not need this eighteenth century relic. Also, being forced to answer to the marketplace by answering to the bottom line, a world of for-profit only hospitals will be able to respond faster to the changing medical environment. Non-profits that are losing money hand over foot will not hang on because of a well-meaning, but financial challenged board of directors. It will motivate hospitals and healthcare systems to find solutions to cost containment. It will spur on medical innovation. Competition in the marketplace works. Plus, all hospitals in the future will have greater flexibility in raising funds and managing their finances that is limited at non-profits, today. To make sure all hospitals in the future function better than they do today, we must remove both the protective barriers and the inflexibility that non-profit hospitals have surrounding them.

I see all of your hands going up out there in objection. I hear the shouts of disapproval from the back of the room. You are saying that it does not feel "right" to eliminate non-profit hospitals. Remember, the rest of the providers of the American healthcare system are for-profit organizations. That includes the pharmaceutical companies, most medical insurance companies, medical laboratories, free standing clinics and urgent care centers, and yes, even your physician's office. Nobody objects to the rest of healthcare making a profit, so we should not do the same to hospitals.

You are complaining that the quality of care will suffer because of the profit motive. Remember, earlier in this chapter we saw that for-profit hospitals, even today, have similar outcomes to the non-profits.

You are worrying that charity work will suffer. Remember, there will be no need for charity work in medicine! Everyone will have healthcare insurance!

Fourth, hospitals will be paid under SPUN by task completed, not time. They will be paid by the diagnosis. It will be based on today's Medicare DRG system. Paying by diagnosis simplifies billing both for the insurer and the provider. Hospitals no longer will have to track every cotton ball they use or aspirin they dispense. Hospital billing departments will shrink. And billing will be one less task for the hospital's overworked, multitasking staff.

Paying hospitals by diagnosis will spur both innovation and specialization. The combination of needing to make a profit plus receiving a set payment for a given patient problem, will encourage hospitals to be creative in curing patients faster, with fewer tests, and more efficiently. In addition, today's hospitals all try to do everything from psychiatric care to childbirth. They are department stores in the era where we need big box specialty stores. Our pay by the diagnosis system will encourage hospitals to pick and choose their strong services that they have enough patient volume. For example, we do not need five medical centers in one city performing heart transplants. Fewer centers doing more volume of specific tasks will decrease costs for the system and improve the quality of healthcare that is delivered.

The payment by SPUN to the hospital for a given diagnosis should reflect its need and value. The problem with today's Medicare DRG payment system is that is underpays for all diagnoses and hospitals must make up the difference with higher reimbursements from other sources. If our dollar amount is a fair one, hospitals will be encouraged both to provide the service and provide it as efficiently as possible. All diagnoses should be weighed on the same scale. There should no longer be ones that are highly profitable, like open heart surgery services, and not profitable ones, like mental health services. This will ensure there is not an oversupply of the profitable ones and an undersupply of the loss creating ones in a given community. The dollar amount per diagnosis will need to evolve over time. Of course, in the beginning, there will be some diagnoses that will not be fairly paid. But those can be identified, and reimbursement quickly corrected. Also, as medical technology changes, the dollar amount paid will reflect those changes.

The beauty of capitalism is that is shifts resources to where they are needed, automatically. Our SPUN payment system for hospitals will do the same thing for health services. An example of such shifting of hospital resources that would occur under such plan would be in the long-term care field. Today, there is a shortage of such resources as they are usually not covered by private medical insurances and Medicare. Since they would be covered on the proposed SPUN plan, the supply would rise to meet this demand in the marketplace. I foresee this demand met by acute care hospital beds that remain in excess capacity, today.

In summary, how the SPUN Healthcare Plan will pay the medical providers and the hospitals will be uniform, universal and simple. This will reduce the administrative costs of providing healthcare in the United States, which is the world's highest as a percentage of total cost. Except for performing procedures and surgery, physicians and other healthcare providers will be paid by time, with a maximum amount of time allotted, based on the diagnosis that is being treated. All time that a practitioner spends with a patient would count as billable time. The system will encourage the use of non-physicians for many clinical tasks and shift the burden of non-clinical tasks to non-physicians. This will ease today's physician shortage and burnout rate. It also will encourage physicians to slow down, not multitask and spend more time with patients. Hospitals, on the other hand, will be paid by task, by diagnosis. This will reduce their billing costs, encourage innovation in treatment and reduce costs in delivering services. The concept of a non-profit hospital will end since there will be no need for charity cases in the future as there will be universal health coverage. The glut in hospital resources will be reduced or will be used to serve resources that are in undersupply today, such as mental health services or long-term care facilities. Such a payment system should paradoxically increase the supply of those health care needs that there is a shortage of today but still reduce the total healthcare costs for the system.

7. HOW WILL WE KNOW HOW HEALTHY WE ARE?

In 1997, a friend of mine, Rick Bartlett told me of a new website that he found. He told me it was called "eBay," and that you could find and bid for almost anything your heart desired. I remembered tying up our home telephone landline (Of course, it was not called a landline back then.) for hours. I remember waiting patiently for just one web paper to load, to slowly load on my computer via my slooooooooooow dialup modem. For those of us of a certain age will remember the awe of the first time they used a modern personal computer. It could have been to send an e-mail to a co-worker across the country or buy something on-line from Amazon and having the item appear on their doorstep in just a couple of days. Maybe it was seeing a picture taken that same day sent from a distant relative or friend. The best part for me was that certain mundane tasks suddenly became a whole lot easier to do. For example, I think few of us sit down and pay our bills each month with a checkbook and a coil of stamps as it is much easier (and saves money on postage) to pay our bills on line. Or even fewer of us pull out folded maps from the gas station to find our way to an unknown destination.

Medicine in general and hospitals in particular, were slow to embrace our modern computer technology. I find this ironic because of all the other high-tech devises that are used in healthcare, today. For we had MRI scanners before we had laptops. We had electronic fetal monitors before we had e-mail. We had neonatal intensive care units before we had cell phones. Let me give you some concrete examples of the dates of this dichotomy. And please remember that I am not particularly tech savvy or the hospital that I used to work for particularly stuck in the 19th century. I bought my first home personal computer in 1994. The first time there were personal computers at my workplace was in 2002. I obtained my first private e-mail address in 1995. But I did not get my first work e-mail address until 2008. I started paying my monthly bills and did my income taxes on my computer in 1996. But it was 2009 before I put down my pen and did my office medical records on a laptop. Finally, until the last day I worked as a physician in 2016, I carried an old-fashioned beeper like the teenagers and drug dealers did back at the start of the twenty-first century.

Why is healthcare slow to embrace today's informational technology? It is because our medical care system thinks like a nineteenth century sail ship designer. He is afraid to walk away from the perfect wooden sailing ship. For centuries, ship design was very conservative. Change was slow coming because a designer knew what worked and what did not. So much was a stake if he made a mistake with a radical change. Therefore, when the nineteenth century rolled around, and it was obvious that steel would replacing wood and steam power would replacing sail, ship design remained in the past and afraid of what obviously was the future.

Medicine, today, is no different. Healthcare workers, in general, and physicians, in particular, are conservative, like our sailing ship designer. We fear change. That includes the radical changes in informational technology. There are other reasons, too. One problem hampering change is that American healthcare systems (hospitals and physician practices) are of a medium size for American corporations. That is, too big to change quickly but too small to afford to rapidly changing technological systems. Plus, healthcare, by its very nature, is a 24/7/365 industry. It cannot shut down its operations (pun intended) for a weekend to install new software on its systems and for a summer to retool its facilities.

Finally, today's practitioners are gun-shy about all informational technology. And rightfully so. Most physicians feel burned by the last attempt by the federal government to push for better informational systems in medicine. This is because of something called "meaningful use." They are two of the most dreaded words that can be heard by a physician, today. Let me give you the background of this tale of woe. In 2009, the United States along with the rest of the world was at the beginnings of the Great Recession. I am sure you remember that because of the housing bubble and debacle that followed it, the economy was slumping, and unemployment was skyrocketing. Congress passed the American Recovery and Reinvestment Act in an attempt to stimulate the economy. It did so by spending money in all areas of the economy. Part of this act was the Health Information Technology for Economic and Clinical Health bill. It encouraged physicians and other practitioners to buy electronic medical record systems (EMRs for short). The federal government gave them incentive payments, if they purchased such systems and if they demonstrated they used such systems in a meaningful way. That latter requirement is the "meaningful use" that I am referring to. There were three stages of meaningful use to show the government that physicians were using their EMRs in a proper manner. Stage 1 promoted the basic use of such EMRs including electronic prescribing of medications. Stage 2 promoted physician communications with each other and patients. Stage 3 promoted better health outcomes. The stages were phased in over the next (this past) decade.

This promotion of electronic medical records was yet another example in the history of American medicine of something that looked good on paper but was a disaster in actual practice. Physicians, as as a group, are cheaper than a free lunch. They rushed out to purchase EMR systems, like it was Black Friday. Their motives were both practical, to improve the running of their practices, and financial, to gain the federal money offered by the incentives. Medical software companies and their salesforce were eager to sell these systems to them. Mostly designed by pimply teenagers who flunked Python, such systems and software were not ready for prime time. Far from it. They were difficult to use. Training was spotty or non-existent. In beginning, especially, they crashed frequently, often shutting whole practices down for hours or days. I remember many a time when I had an office full of patients and the entire computer system would go down. It is not easy trying to give medical care with only having a slip of paper with a blood pressure jotted on it and no other information on the patient. As time went on and physicians had to meet meaningful use requirements to get their incentives, practitioners became fixated on these narrow rubrics needed to meet these goals, often letting actual medical care slip to the wayside. But the real problem was these systems were developed and implemented too quickly without focusing on what should have been their goal, having practitioners give more efficient and better medical care.

But for American healthcare to be efficient and effective, it must follow the words of the great Star Wars philosopher, Yoda, "Train yourself to let go of everything you fear to lose." In other words, American medicine must not be afraid of making quantum leaps in how it does things. Because in informational technology, there is a better way than what exists, today. But to do so, to get there, we must start over again and create an entirely new system of medical informational technology. Let me describe for you what this path would look like for the rest of this chapter.

Online banking is modern marvel. From anywhere in the world, on any computer, or even your smart phone, you can deposit a check, view your account balances and pay your bills. Think about how many different computer systems performing all kinds of different financial functions must come together for this to happen. There are so many different banks, each with hundreds of thousands and maybe millions of users. Yet your money flows seamlessly among them. And it happens, securely and instantaneously. Think of the ease of a computer program like Quicken that can manage all your finances, regardless of how much money you have and how many accounts you maintain and where they are located. With Quicken, at a glance you can see a picture of your financial health.

Guess what folks. Nothing like what we have in our financial world remotely exists for American healthcare. There are many, many different and completely independent computer systems. Let us start at the level of the hospital. There are systems for inpatient medical records, different systems for specialty areas within the hospital like the emergency room or obstetric suite, there are different systems for viewing x-rays and other radiological pictures, there are different systems for tracking medications, and finally there are different systems for billing and finance. Let us now move to the medical office. Again, there are systems for outpatient medical records, but different ones for billing and still a different one for scheduling appointments. Medical data does not flow from one system to another, even within the same organization. For example, a lab test performed in the office does not migrate to the hospital system. Information created and entered in the emergency room in the hospital does not move to the in-patient records.

As we have seen, this makes the practice of medicine in the United States very inefficient. Much of work day for a healthcare worker is spent tracking down missing or incomplete medical information. It does not matter if he is a receptionist in the tiniest office practice or the chief of the medical staff of a major hospital. So much time is spent just logging into one medical informational program after another to find a needed piece of data. Then that piece of data must be copied and pasted back and forth between systems. It is the reason why you are asked the same questions repeatedly as you make your journey through the Disney Land, even for the simplest of medical evaluations.

It is worse than that. Often, we, as healthcare workers do not know what we do not know. Meaning, there is medical information pertaining to a patient "out there" but we do not know that it exists. So, what do we do? You guessed it. We order the same test again. That costs the entire healthcare system money to pay for the unnecessary test and wastes time for the patient and all those involved in getting this redundant work performed.

The answer to this inefficiency is obvious. There must be a single, standard medical records system for *all* parts of American medical care. A universal system for offices and hospitals, acute care facilities and long-term ones, in-patient areas of the hospital and out-patient, general medicine and specialty areas of medicine, even traditional medicine and non-traditional medicine. Is it possible? If they exist in other parts of our world, they can be created for healthcare. There are de facto standards in informational technology that already exist in the business world. All word processing is performed on Microsoft's Word program. Business computers worldwide use Windows as their operating system. Presentations to groups, from kindergarten to the C suite of major corporations, are created and displayed on Power Point. Numbers and statistics are crunched and analyzed on Excel. It does not matter if the numbers are on the laptop of an entrepreneur in his garage or at an oilrig of Exxon Mobil. In medicine, we need a similar standard program for the information we create, use, store and analyze.

It will not be enough that the American healthcare system use the same informational technology programs. All the data must be linked together. If you get a blood test while sick on vacation in Hawaii, it should be displayed on your family physician's computer when you get back home to Philadelphia the following week. Think about it. You can log onto your computer at work to Christmas shop at Amazon and pick up where you left off on your cellphone when you get home. (Do not deny that you shop at work.) The movie you pause on your iPhone's Netflix in the waiting room of your doctor's office can be resumed when you are in bed at night, watching at home. This universal medical data storage system will save time and money for everyone. Time for healthcare workers who now must track down such results and money for the system by reducing duplicate testing.

At its most basic, all medical data will be linked together by the common thread of the patient that it belongs to. That will include the demographic data such as address, phone number, occupation and place of employment. Then, when someone moves or gets a new job, this information will only have to be changed once, not at every medical facility the patient uses. In addition, since there would be just one insurance provider under the SPUN Healthcare Plan, certainly there would be no need to update any insurance information. Or worry if the new insurance will cover the doctors that the patient has been seeing!

All your medical history would be linked together in one file. Every chronic ailment, hospitalization, medication and allergy will be there. There will be no more filling out all those medical history forms when you see a new physician. There will be no more need to update your medication list every time you go to a doctor since all your physicians will have this information, automatically. No longer will you have to try and remember what year you had your appendix removed or what is the name of the little red pill you take twice a day. Instead of having a half a dozen to dozen poorly done and incomplete medical histories scattered about your healthcare universe, you will have a single, complete, always up to date and completely assessable one used by all your health providers.

The dates of all your screening tests and checkups will be included, too. It will be easy to find out when you had your last dental cleaning and checkup or when you had your eyes refracted and examined, last. This basic medical "accounting" of routine care that we all must do will be infinitely easier. Patients and their doctors spend too much time today just finding out when the next routine test or procedure is due. Whether it is a cholesterol blood test, a mammography, a Pap smear, a colonoscopy or a blood pressure check, that information is scattered about. Now, it resides separately in each of those medical providers' files. Or in a crammed folder of dog-eared papers in some drawer in our kitchen at home. Or incompletely entered into our smart phone's calendar. Since no one wants to have any of these tests done just for fun, it leads to these simple tests being postponed or forgotten, making all of us not as healthy as we could be.

Family history among relatives will be linked together, too. Important facts about your medical history can be shared with your close relatives. Knowing whether or not you have hypertension, heart disease, diabetes, certain types of cancer or depression is important information for the medical history of your parents, siblings and children. Today, that information often is not shared, or is shared incorrectly or incompletely. I can recall this occurring on a daily basis when I practiced medicine. When I would take a history from a patient and we got to her family history, the patient often would answer: "My mother had some sort of cancer, but I do not know what kind it was." How frustrating! An opportunity was missed because a medical fact was missing. Of course, under our future system, you will have the choice of what pertinent medical information that you would be willing to share and with whom, to protect your privacy. But I bet, almost all patients would share almost all their health information with their close relatives. After all, we would benefit, in return, knowing what medical conditions, *they* have.

All medical billing systems will be linked together in an ATM-like system. First of all, medical billing, as we have seen, will be much simpler for patients. Patients are only going to be responsible for some occasional co-pays and other modest bills for certain medications. Since all medical providers are going to be linked together through the common entity of the SPUN Healthcare Plan, their billing systems will be linked, too. It will be a snap to pay your outstanding dental bill when you go to the dermatologist. Or pay for your hospital emergency room visit when you go to your eye doctor. Using our PayPal-like system to transfer money, the funds could easily be moved and credited to the right account. Win. Win. You get your outstanding bills paid faster and easier. The medical providers get their money with less time and effort.

Linked and shared medical information will mean much more than saving time and money. It will mean better and complete medical care. For the more accurate and up to date the data that your physician knows about you, the better she can diagnose and treat you. Also, she can spend more time concentrating on what brought you to see her in the first place, rather than chasing down the pertinent facts from your past medical history that is scattered about the healthcare universe.

Not only will all your medical providers have access to all your medical information, so will you. Today, your medical records are treated like that super-secret, "permanent record" from your high school days. You know the one. That record your teachers threatened to change if you did not do what they said. These records are often talked about but seldom seen. As such, your medical records have almost mystical properties attributed to them. They are guarded from our own sight, stored in some faraway vault. And finally, access to them is hard and almost religious in nature.

True, today, some practices and hospitals allow limited access to some of our health information through what are called "online portals." These are internet sites maintained by the individual hospitals and medical practices. The portals allow patients to log onto them with a user name and password. Here, they can access test results, medication lists and summaries of their visits. They remain highly underutilized. I believe that the reason why they are not used very often is that we have too many of them. For example, I have eight separate healthcare portals by my last count. For each portal, it means that burden of trying to remember your user name and password. That is nearly impossible to do for portal sites for physicians that you might only be seeing once a year or less. Plus, when you finally do log on to them, there is a limited amount of information available at the portals, making the effort not seem worth it in the first place.

It is common sense to have one site for all your medical records. Think what tremendous benefits it will brings us! There will be just one site to go and see when and where you had your last eye examination or cholesterol blood test. There will be just one site to find the results of your latest mammogram in a minimal amount of time. Waiting for medical results is stressful, even when they are routine ones. Getting our medical results more quickly will ease that gnawing anxiety of the unknown. There will be just one site to go to find that Latin sounding name for the skin condition that was diagnosed by your dermatologist last year which you forgot the name of.

You will see all the medical information that your physicians see. There will be no more mysterious medical records that are forever hidden from your view. Such an open record system will encourage us to learn more about our medical conditions. Like most things in life, in medicine, knowledge is power. It will encourage compliance with tests and check-ups since it will be so easy to check when they are due. It will foster more trust between patient and practitioner. When records are hidden from view, the air of mystery about them fosters suspicion. There is a feeling that our doctor is hiding something from us or thinks that we are crazy. It feels no different than a locked diary maintained by our spouse. Our imagination cannot help but think it contains the worst. The ability to see what our physician wrote about us and see *all* the information that he sees, will create more trust that is sorely missing in American medicine, today.

The patient access site will be available everywhere there is the internet access, since it will be cloud-based. Smart phone apps will be developed, so patients can carry all of their medical records with them, all the time. This will be so helpful if they become ill on vacation. Parents will have access to their minor age children's records in the same manner, making pediatric care just as open and efficient.

The SPUN Healthcare System EMR will be a two-way street. That is, medical data will flow both ways. Not only will you obtain your medical information, you can enter information into the system, too. You can use the system to schedule your medical appointments. You can use the EMR to order a refill of your medications that will be sent directly to you. Today's technology allows some of this today but requires you to go to multiple sites to accomplish these tasks. Imagine a world where you can schedule your mammography, annual gynecologic examination and refill your oral contraceptive pills all at one website, all in under five minutes!

Your future patient portal will allow you to upload medical data, too. You can enter your weight, blood pressure and heartrate. If you are diabetic, your blood sugars can be entered here. Data from your exercise programs and other activity, gathered by smart devises like Fit Bit, can be transferred here, too. All this data will give you and your physician a moving timeline picture of your health, rather than just a small snapshot of you that she sees in the office. You will be more compliant in doing the things that you should be doing for your health, knowing that it is being evaluated on a regular basis.

The SPUN Healthcare Plan electronic medical records program will have built into it a variety of communications tools for the patient and doctor. Of course, there will be an e-mail application. This will be a simple way for a patient to ask for a prescription to be refilled or for a doctor to let a patient know that a particular medical test came back normal. Second, there will a texting application. Those of you, who are under a certain age, grew up communicating mostly by text. I have watched my Millennial Generation children text their friends back and forth all evening. They will not pick up the phone to talk, like their Baby Boomer father. To improve the under 40 years old generation's communication with their healthcare providers, texting must be a part of the medical record package. Of course, us oldsters will have the option of picking up the phone to contact our doctors directly through the app if we have a question or concern. Finally, there will be a live video option. Think of it as similar to Skype or Apple's Facetime. The eyes are important diagnostic tools in medicine. The ability to see a patient will help the practitioner to help the patient. Many cases where this feature will be useful are obvious. For example, if the patient has a skin rash or a question about her surgical incision, this application would be invaluable. There are some subtle uses of this feature, too. For example, take a physician's evaluation of a patient in pain. A simple glance can judge the severity of the pain and this can be provided by the EMR's video chat feature.

The EMR program's communication features also will allow the same forms of contact among physicians and other healthcare providers. This is more critical than it seems. All the members of your healthcare team must be on the same page when it comes to your health. This is no different than a bunch of different tradesmen building a house. The electrician cannot know when to put in the wiring if he does not know when the house framers have completed their work. Today, medical communications among providers is lacking. It is so bad that the patient often must be the incomplete and inaccurate communicator of such information about her health, back and forth among her doctors. The SPUN program's communications features will enhance the flow of information. For example, a physician will be able to send a text to another physician who is taking care of the patient if she has a quick question or to give the results of her evaluation. Even better, this message will not have to be that detailed. All the medical record information is being shared, automatically. Our video chat feature will be helpful. If one doctor is puzzled by something he is seeing while examining a patient in the office, it will be a snap to get an instant second opinion from a faraway consultant, without anyone leaving their own office.

One of my favorite features about my iPhone is its ability to give me all kinds of reminders. It eases the burden of remembering to do tasks, big and small. Whether it is to be watering the plants, scheduling my car for service, taking out the trash, getting milk when I go to the grocery store or paying my cable bill, reminders make me more efficient and productive. The patient section of the SPUN medical record system will send health reminders to patients, too. Both you and your physicians will have the ability to create these reminders and their parameters. There will be reminders for you to schedule a check-up or health screening, like a needed blood test or dental cleaning. There will be reminders to take your medication, weigh yourself or take your blood pressure. As you check off these reminders being completed, this will inform your doctors that you are being compliant with your course of medical treatment. There will be reminders to keep up your healthy habits. The app will give you a nudge to exercise or drink more water. The reminders will be tailored for each patient's needs. For example, a pregnant mother will receive a daily reminder from the system to monitor her fetus's kicks and movements in the third trimester of her pregnancy.

Health practitioner, too, will receive their own set reminders to make them more effective providers. I look back on my practice years and see this was a critical weakness. It was a case of me not knowing what I did not know. For a physician, today, has no way of knowing information he is missing. For example, if I order a blood test for you, I will get a result in a couple of days. But there is no reminder by the system to let me know that you did *not* go and get it done. I only see test results that *were* performed and *were* reported to me. Too often this led to a tragic comedy of errors. A patient would go and get a critical test performed. Unfortunately, the results were "lost" and never reported to the physician. The patient, not hearing from the physician, assumed the test is normal. The physician, tasked with following thousands of such tests, had no way of knowing the test is lost and abnormal. The final result was the patient suffered from the delay in receiving the information when it finally was reported. It is a major flaw in today's electronic medical records that there are no alert systems built into them for ordered tests that have no results.

Our future electronic medical record system will be capable of giving healthcare workers many more reminders than just missing or pending patient test results. The system will include a notification system for contacting patients for follow up at a particular time. For example, when I did out-patient surgery on a woman, I would contact her, both the day after the procedure and in one week to see how she is doing. If I had a reminder system to tap me on my shoulder, it would become easier to make these calls. Because it would act as a time management solution for all practitioners. It would make our day more efficient, allowing doctors to focus on patient care. To give good medical care, one must be detailed-oriented and compulsive. Most people in the medical field have these personality traits engraved in their DNA. This usually is a major reason why we chose the field. Like the Blackberry of twenty years ago which became the tool that made business people do more, our SPUN EMR should be the indispensable tool for everyone who works in the medical field.

That should be true if the healthcare worker is a physician, dentist, hospital nurse, office receptionist or billing clerk. Even though it will be an all-in-one system, this does not mean everyone's screens and applications will look the same. Just the data will be shared. This is completely different from today where there are separate computer programs for each department and they do not talk to one another. That in turn means that the same pieces of data must be manually transferred over and over again. The goal will be not having to tell a hundred and one people your date of birth and list of allergies every time you have a medical appointment.

Let us look at the features our integrated medical record system will have from the point of view of both the patient and the medical provider. Let us see how it will function from the start to finish of a typical healthcare situation.

The first step in a typical medical encounter is scheduling. Today, that means calling up your practitioner's office or outpatient center to make an appointment. We already have discussed what a pain in the gluteus maximus that is. The phone queues. Being put on hold several times. Negotiating with a rude receptionist for an appointment and hopefully not having to give up a kidney to get one. Not only is it obnoxious, it is enough to turn off many patients from scheduling an appointment at all.

Some medical providers do allow you to make *some* appointments online. The technology is not that difficult as anyone who has made a restaurant reservation with Open Table knows. You may ask why it is not used more frequently. That is because so many appointments are medical insurance dependent. Meaning, whether the future medical encounter will be paid for is dependent on perhaps half dozen insurance variables. Therefore, there is a need for a receptionist to make that determination before they give you an appointment. Simply put, your healthcare provider wants to make sure he will be paid *before* he commits to seeing you. This will be the beauty of a single payer, universal system. All the rules of whether a patient will be seen and what it will cost the patient are the same. And everyone has medical coverage. And with an integrated computer system, the software can inform you of your future out of pocket cost as soon as you make the appointment on line. Therefore, getting 99% of medical appointments under the SPUN Healthcare Program will be as easy as getting a restaurant reservation with Open Table.

Such an online patient scheduling system will extend far and wide from just picking office visits. Think urgent care. Today, when you will walk into such a center with your three-year-old daughter who has a fever and sore throat, you might wait two hours because every other child in your daughter's daycare has the same bug and is there, too. Instead, you will go online and find a nearby urgent care center out of many that has the shortest wait. All the local centers will be displayed like the wait for the popular attractions at Disney Land. You will be able to make an appointment at the center from home, so your child will not have to sit for hours in the urgent care waiting room, infecting everyone else there. This concept can be extended to non-immediate care at hospital emergency rooms, outpatient laboratory and blood drawing centers and X-ray facilities. Perhaps the concept could work so well that we could get rid of most waiting rooms in healthcare. For the very concept of a waiting room implies that the system is inefficient and expects you to wait as you move through it.

One inefficiency in the healthcare system, today, is that too many patients miss their appointments. In medicine such patients are called "no shows." "No shows" represent practitioner's wasted time in a world where there is a shortage of clinician interaction. Added to that is the office staff time and associated cost of tracking down "no show" patients and rescheduling their appointments. "No show" rates from the various studies in the medical literature run from 3% to as high as 80%! (From BMC Health Serv Res 2016; 16:13) A related problem to "no shows" is that of patients who show up for appointments at the wrong time, at the wrong place or on the wrong day. I call these "wrong shows." Patients are "no shows" or "wrong shows" for many different reasons but a primary one is the frantic pace of modern life. Today, practices try to reduce their rate of both by sending out text, e-mail and phone call reminders to patients. (My dentist sends out all three!) There even are automated computer systems that will do this task for practices. Our SPUN Healthcare System EMR will be able to do this appointment reminder function automatically without the need of practice or patient input. Since the future appointment is in the system, it will be a simple software step to have a text, phone call or email reminder sent out to the patient. This will reduce the rate of "no shows" and "wrong shows," and save healthcare practices the cost of either having staff make such calls or paying for systems that make appointment confirmations, today.

The efficiency of a single computer network will extend to when you actually go in for your appointment. Today, the first step when you are at your practitioner's office is called the "registration" process in medicine. You probably call it trying to buy a hotdog from a vendor during the seventh inning stretch of game seven of the World Series and your team is playing the New York Yankees. Translation. It is that huge line of patients waiting in front of an overworked receptionist that you seemingly always see when you enter an office or other healthcare center. And that receptionist is at the same time answering a telephone that never stops ringing. And that line includes people both checking into the office and leaving the office. Plus, it includes an occasional disgruntled patient who has shown up unannounced to dispute a medical bill from the office or a patient who was not able to get through the phone queue there with a medical complaint, demanding an immediate consultation. My "favorite" registration process is at our outpatient center for a local hospital. Here, you wait in such a line, only to find out when you reach the front of it, it is just the "check-in to check in" line. For this line just determines what *second* line you are going to have to wait in to meet with the second receptionist who actually *does* check in for you. Who said the Communist Soviet Union System is dead?

Finally, when you meet the harried greeter at the front of the line, the first thing he does is scan your medical insurance card and driver's license for the hundredth time since you have gone to this practice. (If you want to be stabbed in the back by the people behind you in line, forget to bring either of these items to your appointment.) Next, he shoves a clipboard with a stack of papers at you. It comes with a dried-out ballpoint pen for you to complete the forms. Some of the information asked of you on the forms is reasonable. For example, if you have any complaints, what brings you into the office that day and a review of systems. But most of it is a rehash of what the practice already knows about you. For example, the forms will ask you your address and other demographics, your medical insurance information, what medications you are taking and any allergies. (I am not sure why they ask you for your medical insurance information since they just took a picture of your health insurance card, just ten seconds before.) If there was one set of universal medical records, none of these questions would be necessary. Any demographic changes will be updated at your last visit at *any* medical facility or when you scheduled your appointment online. Finally, there are a bunch of forms for you to sign. You know, the ones nobody reads, and everyone just scrabbles their signature on the bottom of each page. These are medical insurance forms, so the physician will get paid and of course, the universal, tree-killing HIPPA information form.

The registration process should be electronic, simple and short. When you arrive for your appointment, checking in should be the easy process of clicking a few boxes on a touchscreen. This can be done with a portable tablet computer or at an electronic kiosk, like those found for checking into a flight at airports. It could even be completed on your smartphone *before* you even get to the office. Your SPUN Healthcare app on your phone could sense your location and knowing you have an appointment at that time, pop up a reminder to the office that you have arrived. The system will confirm that you are really you with a passcode, or even better, an iris scan or fingerprint scan like found on today's iPhones. The questions the system will ask would be just a few. That is because your health data is up to date, automatically, since it all resides in this one system. These few questions will be tailored to what brings you for that particular appointment. That will get to the meat of your visit, much faster. And the beauty of this proposed system will be that this information will be pass on to all your future visits. For example, you would only have to change your address once, if you should move, even if it is across the country.

Likewise, when the medical assistant calls you back for your appointment, she can concentrate on the medical problem at hand rather than review redundant information. She will gather this information as well as take your vital signs and enter it into her tablet computer or laptop. She will enter it into the SPUN EMR using a screen specifically designed for her medical assistant role. Although everyone using the electronic medical record system is assessing the same data, their view of it will be specifically tailored for them. That is unlike today's systems.

Insurance billers and nurses have the same view of you when they log into a computer, but they need much different information. That should be reflected in *how* it is displayed.

In busy practices, outpatient centers and hospitals, there is a justifiable amount of paranoia about making sure taking care of the correct patient. They want to make sure every patient is receiving the right test or given the right medication. That is why you are asked your name and birthdate a hundred times during every medical encounter. That is why hospitals and some offices give you a wristband with that information on it and scan it when you are receiving a medication or at another critical identification juncture in your care. But there is a simpler and even more secure way to accomplish this verification. The SPUN medical record program will have a built-in scanner of your fingerprint or your iris to identify you at these important care moments. After all, if your Apple iPhone can have this elegant, accurate and rapid identification technology, should not our healthcare system?

When you finally see your practitioner, the computerized medical records program will facilitate the encounter, not encumber it. Again, your practitioner's screen will be unique from what the other members of the healthcare team view, meeting the needs of the practitioner. The view will be different, too, based on *where* you see her. A visit in the hospital room, the emergency room, the office, or at an urgent care center each demand different types of information be readily available to the practitioner. The views will be different based on the specialty of the practitioner. A dermatologist and an ophthalmologist have different medical information requirements to treat you. Today's "one size fits all" electronic medical record systems do not work, just like making all size 10 shoes does not work for outfitting an army. Even within a specialty, informational needs can vary. From my old specialty, I know that I needed different information and wanted to see it in different ways, for my pregnant obstetric patients compared to my non-pregnant gynecologic patients.

The amount of information that the practitioner enters into the system need not be a lot. As we have seen, requiring too much information leads to "cut, copy and paste" medical records. Today's charts are full of inaccurate fluff. Less is more in creating medical information. I remember reviewing some "primitive" paper medical records during my first years in practice. Some encounter documentations were just a couple of lines on an index card. But they were clear and concise. They contained all that was needed for an outside practitioner to quickly understand what was going on with that particular patient in this particular case. A truly useful EMR will guide the practitioner to input just what is needed. No more. No less. As described earlier, the practitioner will be freed from the burden of documenting for the insurance requirements as professional medical billing will be time-based. And this time would be automatically tracked by the system as the patient is being evaluated.

Remember, too, we will have a trained practitioner assistant working closely along with the physician. This new type of healthcare worker can help enter all or most of the information in the electronic medical record for the practitioner.

The computer system will help practitioners practice medicine. Reduced to the very basics, doctors do just two things: diagnose and treat. Using predictive algorithms from the patient's demographics, history and analysis of key words input by the practitioner, the program will suggest possible diagnoses. It will work much like suggestive texts that appear when we input words on our smart phones. As a simple example, if it is February and the program sees the words fever and cough, influenza, as well as pneumonia, would appear as possible diagnoses in the program. (Hopefully even a first-year medical student would have considered these possibilities without the aid of a computer!)

Every so often, a physician comes across a complex case. The diagnosis may not be so readily apparent. The symptoms do not seem to fit together. Such extremely difficult cases will enlist, through the EMR system, both the resources of national experts and the aid of supercomputer problem solving. The latter technology already is being developed with IBM's Deep Blue technology.

In difficult but less complex cases, the practitioner will have the option of getting a consultation right then and there, with the patient. Neither will have to leave the examination room. The physician could chat with the consultant while he reviews the chart on his computer. Everyone will be reviewing the same medical information in real time. This will save the system money and get an answer to the problem much faster. Since the consultant is paid by time, regardless of whether the patient is seen in person or not, he will be compensated for his input on the case by SPUN.

Once the practitioner makes a diagnosis, she picks a corresponding one from the SPUN Healthcare EMR system's database. There will be a limited number of diagnoses to choose from, not the overwhelming number found in today's ICD-10 system. They will be "practical diagnoses." That is, what physicians use when talking with patients and each other about a disease, not the complex insurance-driven ones, seen today. When this diagnosis is chosen, a computer algorithm will suggest further diagnostic tests and treatment options. The EMR will be a partner, silently beside you and your practitioner on your healthcare journey. There will be information on the condition for the patient to read on his version of his electronic medical records. This information will include pictures, diagrams, statistics and links to websites, all designed to inform the patient and make him fully engaged in his own healthcare. There will be information for the practitioner, too. Similar to what the patients sees, but at more technical level as so to better guide the patient's treatment.

After the practitioner chooses the next steps in the management of your hypothetical case, the SPUN Healthcare EMR will make sure it is covered, that is paid for by the insurance system. These determinations will be made automatically by software of the program. With all the needed data entered into the system and having to make a judgement based on only one set of insurance rules, it should not be simple. If the practitioner and the patient decide on a course of management not automatically approved by the SPUN computer, they can appeal to a live person, who is employed by SPUN. Instead of waiting for such preauthorization response coming back in hours or days, it will be made in real time. In a manner like obtaining an on-line consultation, the patient and his physician will appeal via the software on their computer, right then and there. The SPUN arbitrator, a physician with a background and training in the specialty of the patient's problem, will be available for such situations. He will have instant access to all the patient's medical records and can make the decision in the manner of minutes. Having one set of medical records, accessible anywhere there is an internet, makes it all possible with today's technology.

What if you and your physician do not agree with the SPUN arbitrator's decision? There will be a third, higher level of appeal. The case will be reviewed by a physician not directly employed by SPUN. This independent, practicing physician will review the case and make the final determination whether to allow the plan of action to go forward or not. With a standard and universal set of medical records, this appeal process will be much easier and faster than similar appeals that occur today.

Armed with the next steps of the diagnosis and treatment plan, your medical care can move forward, rapidly. If you should need further tests or consultation, the aim would be for those to be performed the same day. You are asking how can such care occur rapidly? First, the scheduling system is integrated. For example, if you are at your family physician and he wants you to see a cardiologist and have an echocardiogram, the family physician's computer can access the cardiologist's and the echocardiogram's scheduling systems and book those appointments, immediately. Second, as we shall see in a later chapter, more medical practices will be vertically integrated. That means a lot of different types of physicians and testing facilities will be all under the same roof. That will make it simple for you just to go down a hallway to have the next step of your diagnosis made or treatment started.

Any needed blood tests will be drawn right then and there. Today, many facilities have the capability to have your blood drawn for analysis at the time of your visit. Primary care physicians commonly have a phlebotomist employed for such tasks. However, with the dozens of different healthcare insurance rules that exist today, many of these insurances do not allow the blood draw at the office. That means, though there is a phlebotomist there, the patient must travel to another facility, go through a second registration process, and wait for the blood draw. What a tremendous waste of time and money! Instead, under the SPUN Healthcare Plan, *every* medical facility will be allowed to be a blood drawing center. For insurance rules should make it easier to get your healthcare, not harder.

The same holds true for any prescriptions you will need. Surprisingly, the actual process of picking up your medications is one area where American medicine has improved a bit over the last decade. Two innovations have made this possible. The first is online pharmacies. For medications you take every day, you get these by mail. This has reduced the number of trips to your local pharmacy, making it more efficient for all involved. The second innovation is the electronic prescribing of medications. This is one (and only) area that today's electronic medical records have made medicine more efficient. For your physician can send you prescription via the internet from her laptop to your local pharmacy's computer system. There, it can be waiting for you when you arrive.

But that still means you must make that trip to that pharmacy. Everyone has had that out of body experience of being sick with the flu, going to your family doctor's office and after being seen, having to make a second trip to the pharmacy, when you are feeling just awful. How can the SPUN Healthcare Plan eliminate that second trip? Healthcare facilities will be able to stock, prescribe and give to you, the commonly used medications used by their specialty. This rule will apply to physician offices, medical clinics, urgent care centers and emergency rooms of hospitals.

The medications will cost you the same wherever you obtain them, whether it be at your practitioner, retail pharmacy or online one. Your practice will stock medications specific for the common, acute illnesses that the specialty sees. For example, in my old practice of obstetrics and gynecology, we saw many cases of yeast and other vaginal infections. Under SPUN, we would be allowed to stock the common treatments for these disorders including Flagyl, Diflucan and vaginal creams. This would save the patient with a vaginal infection that second pharmacy trip for her therapy. "Starter" medications also will be dispensed by your practice. For example, a newly pregnant woman would be dispensed the first month supply of her prenatal vitamin at the office during her first prenatal visit. For the rest of her pregnancy, she would obtain the medication at her mail order pharmacy. That saves her a trip to her local pharmacy for the vitamins as she is waiting for the mail order ones to arrive. And reduce the chance that she would miss those first vitamins early in her pregnancy that are critical for fetal development.

The concept is to create "one stop" shopping for medical

care as much as possible. The easier it is to go for medical care, the more likely patients will seek out care and follow through with treatment. That will reduce expenses in the long run by reducing costs for persistent symptoms due to noncompliance. More importantly, it will make us all healthier.

I hear your complaints. No, I am not crazy. And it is not radical to have providers dispense medications. I am not trying to put my pharmacist friends out of business. First, only a small fraction of medications will be dispensed in this manner. In addition, today's physicians have experience dispensing medications. For example, they stock and dispense vaccines and injections. Also, doctors "dispense" medications in the office by giving out starter samples of drugs given to them by the pharmaceutical companies. The SPUN Healthcare Plan would just expand this concept. Just think about it. No more waiting at your local CVS Pharmacy, with a 102.2-degree fever, cough and headache, for an hour, with everyone else with the same symptoms, for your prescription of Tamiflu to treat your influenza after a visit to the urgent care center. You will just go home and go to bed straight from that center with your medication in hand.

One often forgotten communication barrier in American medicine is language. The United States is a land of immigrants. As such, we have many members of our society who do not speak English. According to a 2015 Census bureau study, one in five or 63.2 million Americans speak a language other than English at home. When a non-English speaking patient seeks medical care, the simple process of communicating her problem moves from complicated to impossible. It creates a terrifying experience for the patient and makes medical care difficult to administer for all involved. Today, the medical profession often relies on a bilingual family members or healthcare worker. Too often, such translators are not available. Some forward thinking hospitals and healthcare systems employ medical translators or use a language line. Language lines are wonderful things. For almost any language, medical translators are available 24/7/365 via the telephone. Some language line systems even have video conferencing technology. It is common sense that our SPUN Healthcare EMR software have this capacity built into it because all Americans deserve adequate healthcare, not just English-speaking ones.

All these innovations in American healthcare would be possible today if we have a universal set of electronic medical records. Information would flow seamlessly between all the centers you go for medical care. Your records from your recent hospital admission will be at your primary care physician when you follow up there in a week. Your dentist will know that you are on a blood thinner without you telling her. Your ophthalmologist will know to look at your retina a bit more closely since you were just diagnosed with diabetes. The need for so many forms, letters and summaries of care will be eliminated as the information would transfer automatically. Physicians and other healthcare workers, today, waste too much time just moving the same piece of information from place to place. With the SPUN EMR software, practitioners will be more efficient by not having to be scribes and concentrate more on patient care.

None of this will happen unless the actual computer software interface is simple, clean, secure and easy to use. Steve Jobs once said during the development of Apple's iPad, that it should be so intuitive to use that not only someone who never used it before should be able to figure out how to work it but also someone who never even used a computer. That should be our usability goal when creating our healthcare system's software. It will so simple to use that anyone who can use a smart phone can figure out the interface.

There are many examples of wonderful hardware and software designs that have this intuitive feel that stand out as possible models for our medical system informational technology. Of course, Apple's iPhone and iPad and any Android smart phone fit this description as pieces of hardware. On the software side, Facebook comes to mind. When you log onto the site, your Facebook "feed" appears. The beauty of it is that from the "feed" you can go so many places on the site. You can chat with a friend through, post a comment for the world to see, look at videos and pictures or "creep" what your children are doing at college beside studying. I have already mentioned the Quicken program for your banking and add to that, TurboTax, for your taxes. Both programs take the dry, complex world of personal finances and make them easy to understand and almost fun, thanks to interactive graphic displays. The Waze app for GPS navigation makes locating and traveling to your destination an interactive game, as well as getting you there as fast and accurately as possible. The Zillow app and website do the same for trying to locate a new house to buy or apartment to rent.

Let us look at what all these designs have in common. All have simple home screen, a graphic rather than a numerical display of data, the ability to see the same information in multiple formats and a sense of fun about them. I am asking the same of the SPUN Healthcare System EMR.

No one wants to use software that when it first loads overwhelms you. That it makes you feel like you just walked from a monk's cell into Times Square in New York City at midnight on New Year's Eve. That is what today's EMRs do to the user. When you first open them, the home screen is overly complex, displays too much information and makes it hard for your eyes to focus on one thing. Instead, the home screen will be simple and welcoming. It will be a basic display of critical information to get the user started.

To accomplish this simplicity, each type of user of the system needs a different opening page. If you are a patient, you want to see a list of your illnesses. (In medicine, we call this your "problem list.") Also, there will be a second list of what medications you are taking and finally an area for alerts. Alerts would include reminders for upcoming appointments, check-ups that are needed, test results that are back for your review and communications from members of your healthcare team. That is all. Nothing else. From here, then you can drill down to the information that you need, such as the last time you saw a gynecologist.

If you are a physician or other healthcare provider, your opening page will be a calendar. You want to see what your day is going to be like. From this opening day planner, you could expand out to see your schedule for the week or month or cone down to see the chart of one of your patients for the day. Like for the patient home screen, there would be an area for your critical alerts and communications.

If you are a hospital administrator's home screen will show how busy your hospital is in its different departments, like the emergency room, obstetric unit and intensive care unit. The concept is that with one quick glance of your homepage, you get a snapshot of what you need to know now to get started at work, without overwhelming you at once with all the details. There are hundreds of different types of healthcare workers in medicine. Each need different summary of information to do their job. Our SPUN Healthcare EMR program homepages will provide that information to them.

I love numbers. In college, I loved the challenge of a particularly difficult integral calculus problem. (No, they are *all* not difficult.) I can spend hours on a budget analyzing my income and expenses in a hundred different ways. I make Excel spreadsheets for almost everything I do in my life. For me, mathematics is the language of God because of the amazing way the universe runs according to equations and formulas.

I realize, though, that this a rare love. Most people do not feel the way I do about numbers and equations. They are a bit intimidated by columns and rows of numbers, or at the very least, their eyes glaze unfocused when they see them. Unfortunately, that is how medical data is presented, today. Laboratory reports from blood and urine studies are represented by long columns of chemical names, followed by a second column of numerical values obtained, a third column of the ranges of normal values, and finally a fourth column if the values are normal, high or low. Ultrasonographic reports of a fetus during a mother's pregnancy have seemingly more numbers, representing different fetal measurements and ratios, than your federal tax return. Records of a hospital patient's weight, blood pressure and other vital signs are just long lines of numbers on a written paper chart or lines on a computer screen. All these numbers tell a story of a patient's health. Today, the story is told in the most unappealing and unrevealing way possible. Because no one pays complete attention to a bland presentation, there is a missed opportunity to extract the most useful medical information.

Let me give you a simple example of how medical data typically is represented and how useful information may be missed. It is from my residency days. A common medical problem is a hospitalized patient who has a fever. If this patient is being treated with an antibiotic for a bacterial cause of the fever, physicians need a way of knowing that their therapy is working. The best way to make this determination is checking that the patient's temperature is returning to normal. However, when a fever breaks, it does not do so in on a nice, straight falling line. It does so with ever so declining peaks of fevers, each peak a little less high than the previous one. This path looks like one taken by a car driving out of the Rocky Mountains. Each mountain that it crosses is lower than the one before until they are just little molehills. (As an interesting aside, most patients' temperatures are highest at night and lowest in the morning, demonstrating our internal biological clock.) During my residency, temperatures were taken by the nursing staff and written in a row across a clipboard. Even today, this method of charting temperatures is most common, except the numbers are entered with a keyboard and represented as a row on a computer screen. My mentor, Dr. Joel Polin, taught me that it was hard to tell if the patient was getting better or not, just seeing a row of numbers. It is difficult to see a pattern in a column of numbers. There is a tendency just to look at the last number to see if it is the lowest on the list. The temperature information is made more useful just by graphing the temperatures versus times. One can see the fever spikes drop much more readily. This gives the medical staff the important information that the patient was improving. Why? Simply put, our brains understand pictures better than numbers. Table 22 is an example of such temperature information, presented in two ways. Which set of data is easier for you to interpret?

Table 22. Two Different Displays of the Same Patient's Temperatures

Date	Time	Temperature
4/27	8:00 AM	103.4
4/27	12:00 PM	102.8
4/27	4:00 PM	102.6
4/27	8:00 PM	102.8
4/28	12:00 AM	103.9
4/28	4:00 AM	103.1
4/28	8:00 AM	101.9
4/28	12:00 PM	101.4
4/28	4:00 PM	100.2
4/28	8:00 PM	101.2
4/29	12:00 AM	101.5
4/29	4:00 AM	100.5
4/29	8:00 AM	99.2
4/29	12:00 PM	99.1
4/29	4:00 PM	98.6
4/29	8:00 PM	100.2
4/30	12:00 AM	100.4

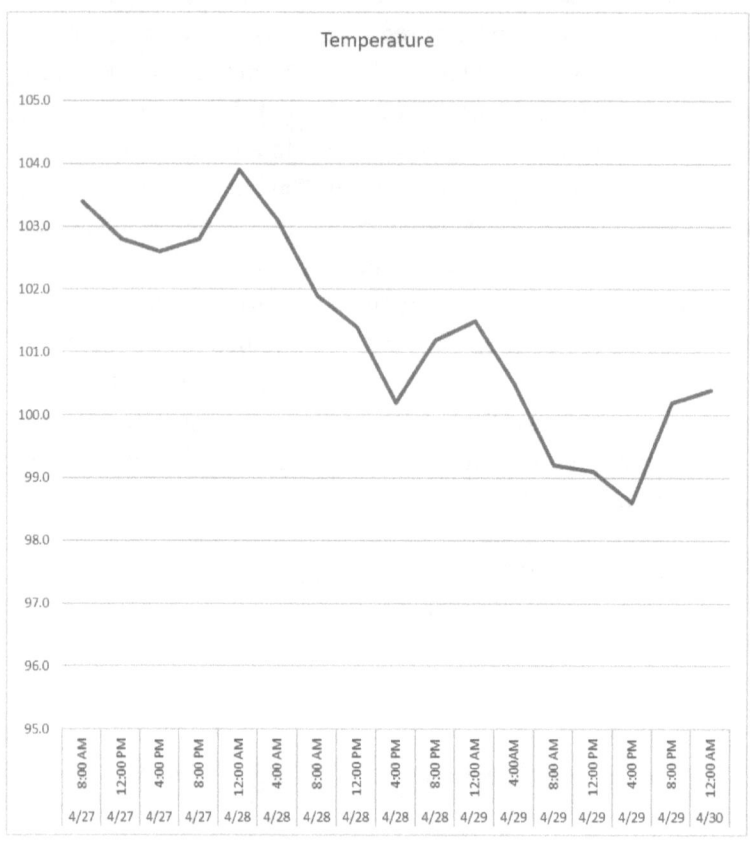

Let us turn our attention to how blood test results typically are reported and how they could be better represented with pictures. Results from clinical laboratories usually are presented in four boring columns, as described above. The only indication that they is an abnormal result is a letter "L" or "H" for a low or high value. Medical professionals want much more information. For example, they want to know how close to normal, the abnormal results are. And if they are normal, where in the normal range they fall. For example, six-foot, one-inch is considered a normal height for an adult male, but it is on the higher end of normal height.

How can our medical record system display this information to the user in a graphic manner? The values can be displayed on a simple line graph with normal parameters marked out. Even a fourth grader is aware of such plots, called box and whisker representations. The box is the range of normal values and the whisker to the wider range of all possible values, including abnormal ones. Merely with a glance of such plots, one can see if a value is normal or abnormal and more importantly, *how* normal or abnormal. Look at Table 23 and see for yourself which display conveys the abnormal results to you best.

We can improve on Table 23. Patients when confronted with lab reports are overwhelmed with all the data that is in front of them. They may panic if they see values out of range. They equate "out of range" with disease. The fix is simple. Let us add traffic light symbols to our laboratory reports. It will be a similar system to our proposed labeling for the health value of our food. These red, yellow and green signals will interpret a list of lab values for the patient (and for physicians, too, since we might see a lab test that we are not familiar with, ordered by another doctor). If all the lab values are normal, the report will get a green light. If there are values out of range but just variations, not indicative of disease, it will get a yellow light. If there was a significant abnormal value that requires follow up, it will get a red light. In addition to the traffic light color, there will be a brief explanation of the meaning of the results and possible causes.

Let us give a traffic light value to the hypothetical report shown on Table 23. That report will get both a red light and a yellow light. The red light is because the white blood count is elevated. The explanation with the red light would say that an elevated white count may be a sign of a bacterial infection, but also can occur in pregnancy or if a patient is taking steroids. The yellow light is on the report because the mean corpuscular volume and the red cell distribution width are slightly out of normal range and almost always of no probable medical significance.

Why did we spend so much time on how lab reports are displayed? Why is it so important that they are reviewed and interpreted in the best manner as possible? First, sheer volume. The typical physician reviews hundreds or not thousands of such reports every working day. Think of a quality control worker on an assembly line making widgets. The more and the faster that widgets that go by, the harder it is to see ones that are not made right. It is easy for medical professionals to have what I call "lab report review fatigue." That is, with so many reports flying by, an important one can be easily missed. Second, the huge volume of abnormal results. For any given test ordered, there is a 5% change that it will come back out of rage. That is because the reference range for normal range is the results for the middle 95% of a healthy control group. That means if there are 20 blood and urine tests ordered, not unusual for typical routine patient testing, one will be out of range. Lab reports need to convey what results are out of range, how far out of range they are and the meaning of being out of range. This will allow the physician to zero in on them. Then he can better interpret what they mean in the context of the individual patient to see if action is required.

Table 23. Two Different Displays of the Same Blood Count Information

Complete Blood Count	Value	Normal Range
White blood count	11.2 k/mm3	4.0-10.0
Hemoglobin	15.8 g/dl	13.5-17.0
Hematocrit	44.7 %	40.0-50.0
Platelet count	165 k/mm3	150-400
Red blood count	4.71 8:00 AM	m/mm3
Mean corpuscular volume	101.1 fl	79.0-99.0
		102.8

Mean corpuscular hemoglobin	31.5 pg	27.0-32.0
Mean corpuscular hemoglobin conc	34.5 g/dl	32.0-35.0
Red cell distribution width	11.3 %	11.5-15.0
Mean platelet volume	11.1fl.	9.0-12.2

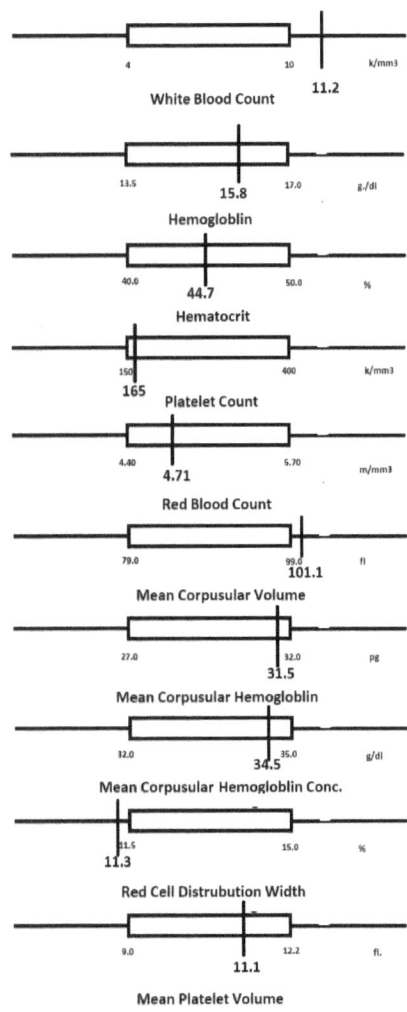

Another way graphic information could better display numerical data is when the same lab test is being repeated. For example, let us say your doctor wants you to be on a low-fat diet because your cholesterol is high. You go for blood cholesterol tests every three months to monitor how you well you are doing with that diet. Your results show your cholesterol is trending downward but there are times there is a small setback. (The vacation to Italy did you in.) Instead of trying to interpret this trend as a list of numbers, printed on different pages or computer screens, there will be a simple graph of your blood cholesterols over time. Like our earlier temperature example, this will better demonstrate this data and how you are doing on your diet.

What can we do about that huge pile of numerical data that a pregnancy ultrasonography generates? When a pregnant woman gets such a scan of her baby, the technologist performing the study takes measurements of different parts of the fetus. These include the head length and width, the head circumference, the abdominal circumference and the length of various bones of the limbs, just to name the most common. After they are taken, the machine also calculates various ratios of these measurements, too. All these numbers are compared to a normal range of values and ratios for the gestational age of the fetus. Abnormal values can be signs of a baby growing too big or not growing enough, important information to have about the health of the pregnancy. In addition, certain abnormal values or ratios of values can be signs of genetic diseases. Typically, these measurements are presented in long and confusing tables, like our blood laboratory report. There is a better way. They should be presented in a pictorial form. There will be a sketch of a fetus with the measurements labeled. Abnormal measurements and the degree of abnormality will be highlighted on the picture. This will make it easier for the obstetrician reviewing the report to understand what is going on with a glance. Plus, it will be an visual aid to educating the parents to be, when they are reviewing the report with the obstetrician.

The same approach will be taken to presenting medical information that is non-numerical, too. This includes radiology reports from x-rays, CT scans and ultrasounds. Also included are pathology reports from analysis of cells and tissue taken from the body. Each specialty has its own studies, too. For example, ophthalmologists review vision tests. Cardiologists have reports from EKGs and cardiac stress tests. Pulmonologists have reports from tests of lung function. Obstetricians have non-stress tests that monitor placental function and the health of the unborn baby.

There will be a simplified diagram or picture of the test results. For example, an x-ray of the hand report would be a simple drawing of the skeleton of a human hand. Any fracture would be represented by an exaggerated break on this cartoon. This approach will point the physician reviewing the x-ray to that area of the hand in either the actual x-ray or the patient's hand. This approach of a simple drawing of the body part being studied with an exaggeration of any abnormality will be used for other x-rays, CT scans and ultrasound studies.

Pathology reports will have a similar approach. There will be drawings and diagrams of the normal cell or tissue structure with an exaggeration of any abnormal structure. I remember many moons ago as a second-year medical student, trying to learn pathology. Everything under the microscope to me looked like a visit to the Museum of Modern Art in New York City. What finally helped me were the pathology drawings by Frank Netter. He was an American surgeon and medical illustrator, noted for his ability to show in simple ways, complex details of anatomy and pathology. His drawings made sense of what I was seeing under the microscope. This approach is needed for all pathology reports. Most physicians and all patients looking at today's reports do not understand what they are seeing under the microscope. To see disease as pathologist sees it takes years of having a trained and careful eye. Simple drawings and diagrams can make sense both of the long Latin words and Picasso paintings of pathology.

This "show it by simplifying it" approach will carry over to tests performed by the different specialists. The results of a vision test would be displayed more than just two numbers, like 20/40. Instead, have a small sample vision chart to *show* what is the smallest line on an eye chart that the patient can read. Or alternatively, *show* how blurry the line is to the patient that she should be able to see. An EKG should be more than just a bunch of wiggly lines and some verbiage interpreting it. The report will show by a combination of magnification and exaggeration *where* the wiggly lines are abnormal and *what* that means about the patient's heart health. The same approach would be used to interpret the wiggly lines in my field of medicine, obstetrics. Our field's wiggly lines are for fetal heart rate monitoring. Fetal monitoring during labor and non-stress tests before, will become more meaningful to those charged to interpret them and less likely to miss abnormalities. Lung function tests should be cartoons of a pair of lungs with the patient's lung capacity compared to what normal volumes should be.

Not only will medical data be graphically displayed to better summarize and interpret it, it should be able to be displayed in several different formats. For example, we should be able to see data displayed over time. One thing I love about smart phone calendars is the ability to zoom in and zoom out in time. I can see what is happening today, and then zoom out to see what is happening this week, this month or this year. Or alternatively, I can zoom in to see what is happening this hour or this minute. SPUN's medical data displays will have that ability. For example, I will be able to zoom out and see what my blood pressure has been doing over the last day, last week, last month, last year, last decade or even longer. For significant changes in blood pressure can develop in any of these time frames, of short interval or long. The same holds true for someone's blood sugars or cholesterols.

The data should be self-annotating for significant events in a patient's medical life. For example, if a patient's insulin dosage has changed, that will be displayed on her blood sugar record to see what kind of difference it made. The same approach will be used for a patient started on a statin for high cholesterol charting, an anti-hypertensive for blood pressure monitoring or the size of a tumor in a patient undergoing chemotherapy.

When the data is pictorial, one will be able to compare it side by side to an older picture, or as a series of pictures. For example, a physician will be able to see two chest x-rays on the same patient, side by side on his computer monitor. A dermatologist will be able to pull up a series of pictures of the same mole of a patient that she has been watching. If an X-box player can have five different game views while playing Halo, medical professionals should have that ability, too.

Which brings us to the last aspect of how the data will be displayed on the SPUN Healthcare System EMR. It must be fun. It should not take itself too seriously. Think about how much fun it was when Microsoft Word, a staid business use program, had Paperclip Man pop up to help you out. Think how much fun it is when you interact with Siri on your iPhone or Alexia on your Amazon Echo. If you have an Apple Watch or a Fit Bit, you know how motivating these watches are to get you exercising. Healthcare workers, from CEOs of large hospital networks to receptionists in small medical offices, will be looking at this program every hour of every working day. Therefore, it should be a pleasant interaction. Thought should be paid to everything, including an eye-pleasing palette of colors. Developers should not be afraid to involve the other senses than sight, meaning the program should talk and interact with you. This does not mean I am proposing a Stethoscope Man or that you will be talking with an assistant called "Elixir" when you are reviewing your blood pressure readings, but there will be an attempt to put a smile on your face when you do use this program.

Regardless of who is providing the information, it will be in the same format for the same type of information. Today, it is very difficult to review medical records from another hospital or another medical practice. Not only are the computers not linked, they display the same information in different formats. When I was practicing obstetrics and gynecology, the different formats made it cumbersome to review a bunch of reports on my patients. Since our Pap smears were read by a half dozen different laboratory, there were six different formats for the results. Ultrasound reports of pregnancies came from twenty or more facilities. Yes, you guessed it. There were twenty different reports. Different report formats, even if there are all formatted well, is yet another set up for missing critical information. Therefore, there will be a universal format for each type of report generated under the SPUN Healthcare Program electronic medical records.

Of course, the medical records must be made secure from hackers. Remember the first time you found out one of your accounts was hacked? How panicked you felt that your financial or other personal information was vulnerable? Now, you probably have what I call "hack numbness" because so many of your credit card, bank, financial, social media and tax records have been stolen since that time. Today's medical records are just as vulnerable. An advantage of designing a system from scratch is making your medical information secure can be a priority from the very beginning rather than trying to put the cat back in the bag after a data breech.

Part of the security for the SPUN Healthcare System EMR will be that information will be on a "need to know" basis. Meaning, everyone in healthcare will not have access to every bit (or byte?) of medical information on every patient. I remember back in the pre-HIPPA 1980s when patient privacy was not a concern, when things were not too busy in the hospital, staff would play "guess how old that co-worker is game." They then would determine the winner from the then primitive hospital computer system. That is because every worker in the hospital had access to every bit of every patient's information. That should have never happened. The best way of preventing such things from happening today is to have layered access to medical information.

You as the patient, will have access to all your information. You also will have access your minor children's records. If someone gives you permission to access some or all their records, you will have access to this information, too. For example, if you have the medical power of attorney for an elderly parent, you will have full access. Or if your sister wants to share the diagnosis of her breast cancer with you, you would have that information added to your medical file, as described above.

A system of user names, passwords or two step verifications will protect your information as you log into the system on your home computer or smartphone. Even better, biometrics like a fingerprint or iris scan will prove you are you and prevent hacking. As mentioned earlier, such scans will be used at each critical point of care as you move through the healthcare system.

When you see new medical providers, a simple click of the mouse will allow you to share your medical information with them. Of course, your medical providers, be it your physician, therapist, medical assistant or nurse would have access to all your information. However, unlike today, when billers and receptionists can view all your intimate medical data, the EMR will limit what information they can see to what is pertinent for them to do their tasks.

It is critical that our SPUN Healthcare Plan EMR have protected and limited access to medical information because there is going to be a lot of data created. Although you may not care if the world knows you had your tonsils removed when you were 5 years old, you probably would care if you have depression or had a sexually transmitted disease. Even such mundane pieces of information like your age and weight are facts a lot of us do not want to share with the world.

However, this data in the aggregate, has enormous yet still untapped potential. Perhaps you have heard of Google Flu Trends. It was a website of Google that estimated how many people have or had influenza in over 25 countries. It did so by looking at how many people used Google search to find out information about the flu. Simply put, the more people that look, the more people have the flu. The intensity of the flu season was reported as minimal, low, moderate, high or intense. Although not perfect, Google Flu Trends achieved up to 97% the predictive accuracy of the Center for Disease Control. Since only summarized data was used, it protected the privacy of those Google users who had the flu.

If Google, a generalized internet search engine, can give us this useful medical information, imagine what data could be mined from the sum of all our EMR records. There is so much that we know that we do not know about health and disease. We could catch the emergence of new diseases. I remember as a fourth-year medical student in 1981, the first time I had about AIDS. The HIV virus, the causative agent of AIDS, was isolated in 1983. But in retrospect, the virus made the leap from non-human primates to humans in Central and West Africa during the 1920s. That sixty-year lag was a missed opportunity to discover and slow the progression and spread of the disease. If a new disease entity such as AIDS emerged today in the United States, there would be a significant but preventable lag to recognize it. Although we are lucky enough in our country to have the Central for Disease Control to help in such discoveries, the CDC is dependent on reporting from individual practitioners and hospitals. With a centralized system of medical records, red flags of new clusters of new signs and symptoms will make the recognition of new diseases easier and earlier.

The same reasoning is true for recognizing the outbreaks of known diseases. As I write this chapter, there is yet another significant and serious outbreak of *E. coli*, passed on by romaine lettuce. Whether the food-borne illness is caused by *E. coli*, salmonella, or listeriosis, it is critical to find the food source. A universal and complete national set of medical records will make it much easier and reduce the impact of the outbreak. Think the yearly flu season. Some winters see more influenza cases than others. Because there is not universal set of medical records, not all cases are reported. Knowing the true incidence of influenza and where it is occurring will help drug companies that make flu anti-viral agents and influenza test kit manufactures. It will alert practitioners in high outbreak areas to look out for the disease.

It is important to know not only that diseases are occurring and how many cases they are, but also *who* is getting the disease. Because knowing what risk factors cause a disease may lead to ways to prevent it. Take cigarette smoking. Tobacco use was common and widespread in the United States, before the country as such existed. But it was not until the 1930s that a tentative link was seen between cigarette smoking and lung cancer. And it was not until 1964 that there was enough evidence for the Surgeon General of the United States to issue his report detailing the link. Think of the hundreds of thousands of lives that could have been saved if we had known sooner. We do not know the causative factors of most diseases. For example, we are not even sure what kinds of diet are linked to higher or lower risks of heart and other cardiovascular diseases. Having a huge national database would be a big step forward to understanding and preventing many diseases. Such a database will contain every single affected patient. More importantly, such a database would have every piece of health information on that patient to find such an association.

A national database will be a gold mine in finding better tools for diagnosis. All medical tests have an associated rate of false positives (Patients whose tests are abnormal but do not have the disease.) and false negatives. (Patients whose tests are normal but have the disease.) Both are terrible ordeals for patients. Patients who have false positives must go through more testing which leads to worry, pain and possible complications from such testing. Patients who have false negatives are lulled into a false security that ends when they are hit in the face with the diagnosis. Surprisingly, we do not have the answer for the best ways of screening and diagnosing many common and serious diseases. For example, the parameters for the diagnosis of hypertension have just been made more stringent. The type and frequency of screening for the common cancers of the breast and of the prostate continue to be reviewed and revised. The type of testing for precursors of cervical cancer, called dysplasia, are in flux. Data mining the medical records of the SPUN National Healthcare System will answer hundreds of questions such as these. Having the best diagnostic tools means lower costs to diagnosis, less anxiety from false negatives and false positives, and a healthier population.

If a national database is a future gold mine for diagnosis, it will be a diamond mine for treatment. One of the rituals of medical school is a speech all students receive during orientation. New students are informed that half the information they will learn over the coming four years will be wrong by the time they graduate. And to make matters worse, no one knows what half of the information is the wrong half! This evolving change of medicine especially is true when it comes to treatment. Therapies that are the standard of care today are discarded and replaced, tomorrow. Only part of the reason is because new treatments come alone. Just as often we find our current therapy is useless or harmful. To find the best possible therapy, whether it be a cancer or a common cold, required data and lots of it.

With a national database of every possible diagnosis and having the results of different treatments, medicine can get at these answers sooner, so we all can be treated more effectively with less complications and live healthier lives.

Part of me is a Mary Poppins optimist. I believe that the many of the answers that medicine has been searching for since the beginning of time, such as the causes and cures of cancer, exist today. They just must be mined in the data we already have. Looking for these answers in one mine rather than tens of thousands will get us these answers a lot sooner.

I also am an optimist that such a universal medical record system having the criteria that I have described can be created, today. For I see no giant leaps of technology that must be made. All the software, hardware and cloud tools for such a system exist today. I am most hopeful that it can take place because of what we have as a nation to draw upon to make it happen. Think of Apple, which has created intuitive products, such as the iPhone and iPad. Think of Google which has organized the entire Internet and made it accessible with the click of a mouse. Think of Microsoft which has put a computer in every school, business and home. Think of Amazon which has made Cloud computing a household world. With resources such as these, creating and maintaining such a medical records system will be a snap. I challenge Jeffery Bezos, Mark Zuckerberg, Bill Gates, Tim Cook and anyone who would like to emulate them to this critical task for our country's health.

8. THE FIRST THING WE DO, LET'S KILL ALL THE LAWYERS

Every physician has his favorite medical malpractice story. Gather a group of doctors together at a social event, and each will try to top the rest with his ludicrous liability tale. It is not unlike a group of fishermen trying to outdo the rest with a story of the "one big one that got away." I am sorry, dear reader, but please indulge me by letting me tell my story. When I was in my first year of obstetric practice, I was faced with a complicated and challenging delivery of a set of twin babies. Early in the mother's labor, the father of the baby made sure that everyone in the obstetric suite knew that both he and his wife were attorneys. This, by itself, is a common occurrence for medical workers. People think that namedropping or revealing their profession is like slipping the hostess of a restaurant a twenty-dollar bill to guarantee a good meal. But its effort is the complete opposite. It is more akin to an opposing football team calling a timeout just before a field goal kicker is attempting the tying score with time expiring in a championship game. Common sense says that adding more pressure to a pressure-filled situation does not improve performance. Back to my story. Then, right as I was scrubbing for the twin delivery, the father stood toe to toe with me, with his jugular veins of his neck bulging. He then threatened me with the scream: "If you hurt one hair is on either my babies or my wife, I'll sue you for everything you have, doc!" Luckily, everything went fine with the delivery. Both babies and their mother did great. And the husband did apologize to me after the fact.

I tell you this tale to help you understand what is feels like to practice medicine in the United States under our present liability system. It does not matter if you are a physician, nurse, orderly or CEO of a hospital. The system puts the constant fear of failure in our conscious mind for every professional action we perform. Despite the title of this chapter, I do not hate lawyers. As the saying goes, some of them are my best friends. They are no different than any of us. They are working hard, trying to pay their bills and hope to send their children to college. But I do blame the system, in this case, the American tort system. For it is a major culprit in what is broken in medicine, today.

Let us explore how we got ourselves into this mess. Torts are part of civil law. That is, a separate legal system from criminal law. Civil law is about individuals doing bad things to others in a society and addressing compensation to make up for the bad thing, Criminal law is about individuals doing bad things against the society and addressing punishment for the bad things. Think back to the infamous O.J. Simpson case. He was found not guilty of murder in his criminal case but lost his wrongful death lawsuit in the civil case.

The differences between the two legal systems are significant. Criminal cases can only be initiated by the government, called in such cases, the prosecution. Civil cases can be initiated by anyone, called in these cases, called the plaintiff. In criminal cases, the prosecution must prove that the defendant is guilty "beyond a reasonable doubt" while in civil cases, the plaintiff only has to prove that the defendant is liable by a "preponderance (or majority) of evidence." Defendants in criminal cases have more constitutional rights than in civil cases. Finally, for criminal cases, the jury must decide a unanimous verdict while a simple majority rules for a civil case.

A tort is the legal name for the wrong one person does to another, whether intentional or not. If you trip on my broken sidewalk, or if I smash into your car in a traffic accident, I have committed a tort against you. Medical malpractice is a negligence type of tort. Negligence means carelessness in this context. To be judged negligence, the action must meet the criteria of what lawyers call the "four Ds:" duty, dereliction, direct cause and damage. "Duty" means the person taking care of you have an obligation to do so because of an established physician-patient relationship. "Dereliction" means the injuring party did not do their duty and this is judged by what is called the "standard of care." That means physicians and other healthcare workers are judged by what is typically done by their peers in that particular medical case. "Direct cause" means that the dereliction led to the injury. That means something that the healthcare workers did or did not do was the prime cause of the tort. Finally, there must be "damages" or injuries. Such damages can be psychological and financial as well as the obvious physical ones.

Let us take a simple and obvious example of a medical malpractice tort. An orthopedic surgeon amputates the wrong leg of his patient. This would be judged malpractice because (1) the surgeon had a duty to take care of the patient, (2) he was derelict in not meeting the standard of care of operating on the correct leg, (3) he directly caused the injury as his surgery was on the wrong leg and (4) there was obvious physical and other damages caused to the patient by the wrong amputation.

An important concept of medical liability is the medico-legal theory of "informed consent." At its most basic, it obliges the physician to tell the patient the risks of a medical procedure or other therapy. The theory is that the patient then can weight its risks versus its benefits, the pros and the cons, in making her decision. Remember nothing is as simple as it appears in American medicine. What is both common sense and good ethics on paper is a nightmare in the real world. Informed consent is a yet another example of something that should build a relationship between the healthcare partners of patient and physician, but instead adds more bricks to the Berlin Wall separating them.

I am not saying that patients should be blind and uninformed to what is going on with their medical care. This, unfortunately, was too often the case, less than a generation, ago. But medicine is complex. It is much more complex than patients realize. It makes it difficult for physicians to simplify the nature of illness and disease to patients and their families. It can be best likened to a theorical physicist explaining quantum mechanics to a seven-year-old. For there to be true informed consent would require sending the patient to medical school for four years. Today in medicine, there are unanswered questions about how much detail is enough detail. How rare must a complication be that it can ignored in the explanation to the potential patient. For example, I knew an obstetrician-gynecologist who taught a mini-medical school course every time she obtained an informed consent for even the simplest of surgeries. I overheard her once going over with her patient the risks of a D and C. "D and C," short with dilation and curettage, for those of you who might not know, is a diagnostic surgical procedure where the woman's cervix is opened, and the lining of the uterine wall is scraped to obtain tissue for examination. An uncommon complication, with about one percent risk, is that a hole may be accidentally made in the wall of the uterus. In such cases, a laparoscopy is needed. A laparoscopy is a second, more involved operation that looks inside the abdomen through the patient's bellybutton. It is needed in such cases to make sure that there is no bleeding or organ damage from the hole made in the uterus. Of course, it is reasonable to inform a patient who is going to have a D and C performed about this risk. But my gynecologist friend would spend additional half an hour going over all the possible surgeries that might be needed if something was found at the laparoscopy. And then go over all the risks of complications of *those* surgeries. And so on and so on. Such a litany just scared the poor patient. Even worse, it built a wall a distrust between the surgeon and the patient.

Some practitioners try to simply this process of informed consent by giving out handouts, booklets, showing videos and even videotaping their encounter with the patient. All these maneuvers are full of good intentions. But most patients find the whole process overwhelming at a time in your life when you already are overwhelmed. Remember the last time you bought a house and were at its closing? Dozens of papers were shoved at you for you to sign. You knew you were signing your financial life away, but you just signed them anyway, knowing you would not get your new house, otherwise. That have been my experience with my patients. Almost all patients, even lawyers, just sign the informed consent forms without even reading or understanding them, knowing that is only way they are going to get the surgery or procedure that they need.

The SPUN Healthcare Plan can solve this problem of uneven and overwhelming informed consent. It will standardize the process. For each medical procedure, from the simplest skin mole removal to a liver transplantation, there will be an informed consent created for the system. It will be an interactive, visual explanation of the nature, pros, cons, benefits and risks of the procedure in non-medical terms. It was be part of the electronic medical record so the patient will have access to it, anytime and anywhere. Being standardized across the country and developed by medical writers and medical practitioners, it will ensure there is enough but not too much medical information provided for patients. It will not overwhelm them and not interfere with the relationships with their physicians.

There are other problems with informed consent as it exists, today. What do you do in cases of minor children or incapacitated adults? How about in emergency cases when no one with a medical power of attorney is available to provide consent? Because informed consent is so tied up with medical liability rather than patient education, physicians today view it as a time to CYA. Therefore, common sense typically disappears in these cases. To solve these problems, we must solve the liability problem. That will return informed consent to its original role of educating the patient, building rapport and trust, and a positive professional interaction.

Suing for medical malpractice goes back to the dawn of history. Have you heard of the infamous saying: "An eye for an eye?" That statement comes from the Babylonians, composed in 1794 BC. It was part of the Code of Hammurabi, the first written laws in the world. It means medical practitioner would for punished for his medical mistakes. In this case, a rather harsh one for a physician who injured a patient's eye during treatment. In the same vein, (no pun intended.) the ancient Greek Hippocratic Oath preached to physicians to "At first, do no harm." That is, doctors should avoid mistakes in practice.

Tort law in the United States was borrowed from abroad. Our country took our legal system from the English. When we study English law, we find the first legal case of medical malpractice was in 1374. In the case of Stratton v Swanlond, Agnes Stratton and her husband sued her surgeon, John Swanlond for not properly treating her injured hand. Surprisingly, the surgeon won on a legal technicality! The term, "malpractice," was coined by the famous English legal scholar, William Blackstone in his 1765 "Commentaries on the Laws of England." He based the name on the Latin words "mala praxis," meaning bad practice.

The first medical malpractice lawsuit in the United Sates

occurred in 1794. The plaintiff won a verdict of 40 pounds against the surgeon who operated on his wife, causing her death. Before becoming the sixteenth president of the United States and leading our country at the time of the Civil War, Abraham Lincoln was a medical malpractice lawyer both for plaintiffs and defendants.

The late nineteenth century saw the legal pendulum swing toward the plaintiff in malpractice cases. People were becoming less fatalistic in their personal philosophies and were less likely to interpret bad outcomes as just "God's work." Even today, more conservative areas of the country tend to favor the defendant more often than in more liberal ones. Also, the thanks to such steps as the formation of the American Medical Association in 1847, medicine was becoming more professional. Therefore, expectations of a good outcome were higher. Liability insurance, to cover medical malpractice cases, came into being in 1919. The Massachusetts Medical Insurance Society was the first such insurer in the United States.

Medical liability became a problem in the United States during the 1960s and 1970s. Both the number of lawsuits and the size of the verdicts grew in leaps and bounds. Let me give you just one statistic to show the enormity of the problem. In the United States, today, there are 15 medical malpractice lawsuits filed every year for each 100 physicians. There was no one cause for this problem. The events of the decade, such as the Vietnam War and the Watergate Scandal made the country, in general, less trusting and more cynical of those in authority. Medicine became expensive, complex and impersonal. It is much easier to sue some huge hospital corporation. It is not hard to sue a rude physician who you only encountered for five minutes and you never met before or saw afterward. That is much harder than filing a lawsuit against your family physician who you have known your whole life, is your neighbor and child's soccer coach. Most physicians now carried medical malpractice insurance. This creates the perception of "deep pockets" that will pay on all claims that are made. Liability lawyers aggressively market themselves on the television, radio and in newspapers. Potential plaintiffs see no risk for yourselves in creating a claim since such lawyers work on a contingency system. This means they only got paid if they won the case. Typically, it is a percentage of the settlement. It feels like playing the lottery. We live with that legacy from fifty years ago, today. Although many states legislated some minor reforms to the system, medicine remains a highly litigiousness field.

Let us now examine today's medical liability system. Let us define what its purposed should be and if today's system accomplishes them. Its first goal is compensating patients who have been harmed by medical errors. According to a famous study from Harvard (Harvard Medical Practice Study. A report of the Harvard Medical Practice Study to the State of New York. Cambridge, MA: The President and Fellows of Harvard College; 1990. Patients, Doctors, and Lawyers: Medical Injury, Malpractice Litigation, and Patient Compensation in New York.), it fails miserably. For only one patient in 15 who was harmed because of medial neglect ever received a settlement. Why do so few injured patients receive a settlement? Many have medical or disability benefits that cover their costs of the injury. Some patients do not want to antagonize their physician who they may still trust and want to continue to see. Americans, in general, do not have a high regard for the legal system or trust lawyers. Many cases are so minor that lawyers will not take them as it is not worth their time and effort. Remember, they are paid as a percentage of the claim. Finally, and perhaps most important of all, many patients remain in the dark, not knowing that medical malpractice occurred.

In our bizzarro medical world, the opposite also is true. According to the Harvard study, five-sixths of patients who received compensation had no evidence of negligence. Why does this happen? The legal system, as it stands today, is an imperfect judge of the quality of medical care. Defense and plaintiff lawyers vary tremendously in quality. Smaller but defensible cases may be settled rather than generate large legal costs to defend. The small number of cases that go to trial are decided by a jury. The jury's decision need only be based on a preponderance of the evidence and just by a majority of the jurors. Jurors have a difficult time understanding the nuances and complexities of medical care. Plus, they carry with them their own prejudices based on their own experiences with the healthcare system.

To make matters worse, patients do not receive even half of the money spent on medical liability. According to a study published in the New England Journal of Medicine in 2006 (Studdert David, M, Mello Michelle M, Gawande Atul A, Gandhi Tejal K, Kachalia Allen, Yoon Catherine, Puopolo Ann Louise, Brennan Troyen A. Claims, Errors, and Compensation Payments in Medical Malpractice Litigation. New England Journal of Medicine. 2006;354(19):2024–2033.), only 46 cents out of a dollar spent on medical malpractice insurance goes to patients as compensation. The rest goes to pay the legal expenses of pursuing and defending such cases, the court systems reviewing such cases, and the expenses of the malpractice insurance companies. Look at it another way. The overhead to compensate injured patients is more than the payments, themselves. And this is assuming that all patients who received payments had a justifiable claim. I am not arguing that patients who had preventable harm done to them not be compensated, but there must be a more efficient way than with our present tort system. My logic? Most patients who are harmed by a medical error are not compensated. Most of those who are compensated were not harmed. Most of the money spent on medical malpractice does not go to the victims. We must conclude that our medical liability system fails at its primary goal of compensating patients that have been harmed.

The second goal of any medical liability system is the threat of a malpractice suit should make healthcare safer. It should weed out practitioners and hospitals that practice bad medicine and reduce the occurrence of such events. Unfortunately, today's system fails at this goal, too. For the evidence shows this is not the case. First, medical injuries are way too common. That implies practitioners can do much better, despite the threat of a lawsuit. A study of hospital admissions in New York State (Brennan Troyen A, et al. Incidence of Adverse Events and Negligence in Hospitalized Patient: Results of the Harvard Medical Practice Study I. New England Journal of Medicine. 1991;324(6):370–376.), found that in 3.7% of cases, a patient had an iatrogenic injury and a quarter of those were the result of negligence.

This study is confirmed by Johns Hopkins experts who studied data over eight years. They calculated that over quarter million deaths per year in the United States are due to medical error. If it were listed as a reportable cause of death, it would rank number three. Some researchers claim even this number is conservative. They feel perhaps one million deaths per year are due to medical mistakes. Table #24 summarizes the depth of the problem. It lists the incidence, deaths and dollar cost of specific medical errors per year, based on different studies. For every time you go into a hospital as a patient, there is a 2.1% chance of a serious drug reaction, 5% chance of getting a hospital acquired infection, 4 to 36% chance of having an iatrogenic injury and a 17% chance that there will be a procedural error performed on you. These errors are due to poorly coordinated patient care, fragmented insurance networks, missing safety net systems for patient care and lack of accountability of physician practice. These are system failures. But do not be surprised. How could there not be system failures because we do not have a real medical care system in this country?

Table 24. Annual Death Rate and Costs of Medical Errors by Cause in the United States

Medical Error	# Deaths/Year	Cost ($ Billions)
Adverse Outpatient Events	199,000	77
Bedsores	115,000	55
Malnutrition	108,800	
Adverse Medication Reaction	106,000	12
Medical Errors	98,000	2
Iatrogenic Infections	88,000	5
Unnecessary Surgeries and Procedures	37,136	122
Surgical Related Complications	32,000	9

Second, as we have noted, most cases of medical negligence do not result in a lawsuit. And most settled lawsuits are not the result of medical negligence. Therefore, our system is like poor parenting. Image if you disciplined your seven-year-old child once week when he is just doing his homework, but you let him get away with fighting with her sister and not taking a bath. Do you think he would learn the right way to act? Out medical liability system fails to reduce medical errors because legal actions are not correlated to them.

Third, there is a long delay from the injury through the start of a malpractice suit to its resolution. Unlike an episode of LA Law, the American legal system works ever so slowly. On average, it takes 2 to 4 years for cases to reach their conclusion. A decade or more time is not unusual. This long, legal case timeframe has several detrimental effects. It slows the time for the injured party to heal emotionally, as there is no immediate resolution. For the defendant, it unlinks the connection between the event and the "punishment." This negates any possible learning from the mistake or effecting a change in practice. To follow my analogy above, you cannot punish your child 2 to 4 years after he broke your china vase playing baseball in the dining room and expect it to stick.

Fourth, medical malpractice insurance is not like your auto insurance. If you are in a bunch of car accidents, your rates will skyrocket, or your insurance company may drop you, entirely. Medical malpractice insurance rates are not highly correlated with a physician's claims history (Sloan Frank A. Experience Rating: Does It Make Sense for Medical Malpractice Insurance? American Economic Review. 1990;80(2):128–133). Therefore, even if there is a truly poor performing physician or hospital that has a lot of medical malpractice lawsuits against them, it is not going to financially prevent them from continue to (mal)practice.

So far, we can conclude our present medical liability system does not reduce medical errors and does not fairly compensate victims of medical negligence. It is even worse than that. For not only does the system not do what it is supposed to do, it has additional toxic effects on the rest of the American healthcare system. The fear of a malpractice suit psychologically teaches physicians and other medical caregivers to practice defensive medicine. The randomness of such liability suits creates mass paranoia. Practitioners become like a child that is punished unexpectedly when he does nothing wrong. For the fear of "getting sued," unfairly is never far from the mind of anyone in the healthcare field.

Let me give you a common "behind the scenes" example. So many conversations among health personnel follow this script. It begins as a debate about what is the best step to take in the treatment of a certain patient, Joe. Dr. Mike will argue to follow path "A" to treat Joe. He bases his decision on empiric data from the medical literature. Dr. Mike, typically, is a neophyte, such as a resident or young attending physician. Dr. Mike's idealism and naivety is quickly shot down by Dr. Pete.

Dr. Pete argues for a more aggressive and expensive path "B." Dr. Pete agrees that the textbook "A" solution would be the best answer on a written test. But in the real world, to prevent from being sued, the team should follow path "B" to treat Joe. Dr. Pete, being older and higher up the medical command chain eventually wins the argument. Path "B" wins the day. I do not know how many marginally indicated cesarean sections I saw performed under such circumstances. Or how many expensive and unnecessary CT scans, ultrasonograms and MRIs I saw ordered, with their inherent risk of radiation exposure and finding of a false positive incidental finding that led to even more tests and created so much patient anxiety. Or how many patients were admitted to the hospital who did not need to be there, "just to be sure."

For "just to be sure" are the most expensive, anxiety producing and dangerous words in medicine. They create the false perception that everything and anything is being done for the patient. They are a script for a potential malpractice jury a decade in the future. For the words state that the healthcare team was "all in" despite the eventual poor outcome. However, these situations are no different than the police officer who uses excessive force at a traffic violation stop. Because in both cases, those in charge are being overly aggressive. "Just to be sure" always is the more expensive path. But since neither the patient nor the physician is directly paying for the care, it is not resisted on financial grounds. "Just to be sure" always is the more anxiety producing course of action. The more tests and more procedures recommended to a patient heightens her concern that the situation is worse than it really is. Trusting the physician's judgment, the patient becomes caught up in the group paranoia, too. And ironically, "just to be sure" is the more dangerous path to follow. All tests and procedures have inherent risks. By trying to be "too safe," doctors create more chances for danger.

You may be asking for proof that doctors practice defensive

medicine. You may say that my tirade is the expected reaction of an obstetrician-gynecologist from a large metropolitan area of the country. That is, someone in the very highest medical malpractice risk specialty in a high liability area. Let me show you. First, let us define the term "defensive medicine." It is the doing or not doing things in practice of medicine that are not beneficial to the patient but serve to protect the practitioner from future medical liability. Defensive medicine come in positive and negative forms. Positive, by far, is most common type. It is the ordering of extra tests or supplying extra therapy that are not needed, have been shown to be not cost effective and have no benefit for the patient. Negative defensive medicine also takes place. It is the refusal to do care that could help the patient out of fear that there may be an adverse outcome and the resultant lawsuit that might follow.

The first evidence that there is a lot of defensive medicine practiced in the United States today is from surveys of physicians. In 2004, researchers (Studdert David M, Mello Michelle M, Sage William M, DesRoches Catherine M, Peugh Jordon, Zapert Kinga, Brennan Troyen A. Defensive Medicine among High-Risk Specialist Physicians in a Volatile Malpractice Environment. JAMA. 2005;293(21):2609–2617.) simply asked 824 physicians from high risk for medical malpractice suit specialties (emergency medicine, general surgery, orthopedic surgery, neurosurgery, obstetrics and gynecology, and radiology) in Pennsylvania whether or not they practiced defensive medicine. Almost all, 93% of the surveyed group, answered yes. The surveyed physicians admitted to both positive and negative defensive medicine. Positive defensive medicine was more common, 92%, and included the ordering of unnecessary tests, the performing of unneeded diagnostic procedures, the trite referral to another specialty practitioner, and the clinically unnecessary use of radiologic testing. Negative defensive medicine behaviors were seen in 42% of physicians. This included the elimination from the practice of high liability procedures, avoiding patients with complex medical problems and those perceived as litigious.

You may argue that all physicians are cynical like me (and they are). That they answered surveys that way, even though in reality, they do not practice defensive medicine. Where is the proof that defensive medicine truly is being practiced because of medical liability? Such proof comes from a comparison of medical practices between high liability and low liability states. The laws governing the conduct of medical malpractice cases are created at the state level. These laws vary from state to state. Some favor the plaintiff, the alleged injured patient (high liability states) while others favor the defendant, the physician, medical practitioner or hospital (low liability states). Low liability states have instituted laws that have put caps on the total claim that can be paid out, caps on the "pain and suffering" portion of the claim or made it more difficult to file a suit by requiring a certain amount of expert opinion from physicians before it can be started.

Hellinger and Encinosa made such a comparison study in 2006 (Hellinger Fred J, Encinosa William. The Impact of State Laws Limiting Malpractice Damage Awards on Health Care Expenditures. American Journal of Public Health. 2006;96(8):1375–1381.). They found low liability states have between 3 and 4 percent less overall health spending per capita than states that do not. This has been confirmed in a study by Baicker and associates in 2007 (Baicker Katherine, Fisher Elliott S, Chandra Amitabh. Malpractice Liability Costs and the Practice of Medicine in the Medicare Program. Health Affairs. 2007;26(3):841–852) who found there is a direct association between higher medical liability premiums and jury awards and how much is spent per capita on a Medicare patient.

Where does the extra medical spending in high liability states go compared with low ones? The same Baicker study answers this question, too. It is on advanced imaging studies, like CT scans and MRIs. This is not surprising. Remember earlier when we said that the one area that the United States leads the world is in such spending per person. Now, we have a reason why, the effect of our medical liability climate on creating more defensive medicine.

Defensive medicine not only costs the system more, it leads to worse medical care and outcomes. For example, studies show that it leads to a higher rate of cesarean sections among birthing mothers but without an improvement in birth outcome. (Dubay Lisa, Kaestner Robert, Waidmann Timothy. The Impact of Malpractice Fears on Cesarean Section Rates. Journal of Health Economics. 1999;18(4):491–522) The researchers found this effect by looking at birth certificates from around the country. In particular, they looked at the cesarean section rate in low malpractice premium counties versus high ones. The high premium ones had a higher rate of cesarean sections but without better outcomes for the mother and baby.

How significant is this effect? The rate of cesarean sections in the United States was 5% in 1970, rose to 20% in 1970 and was 32% in 2015. Experts say an ideal rate should be approximately 19% of all births. Stop for a second and think about what that means. There are about 4 million births in our country each year. That means 32% minus 19% of those American mothers or 520,000 each year pay the price of our bizarre medico-legal environment with scars on their bellies and unneeded pain and suffering from surgery they did not need. They and their babies also suffer the short term and long-term effects of not having a vaginal birth.

Our liability system's flaws affect the prenatal care side of obstetrics, too. In areas with high malpractice premiums, prenatal care starts later in pregnancy and there were fewer visits per mother than in low ones. (Dubay Lisa, Kaestner Robert, Waidmann Timothy. Medical Malpractice Liability and Its

Effect on Prenatal Care Utilization and Infant Health. Journal of Health Economics. 2001;20(4):591–611). I picked obstetrics because it was the branch of medicine that I practiced for 34 years and therefore, have the most familiarity. But I easily could have picked another specialty because other studies show similar results.

So far, we have found our malpractice system does not compensate the right victims, does not even spend most of money on them, does not prevent bad medicine, and leads to unnecessary and sometimes harmful defensive medicine. The next question we ask is how much does it cost us in dollars and cents for having such a malfunctioning medical liability system. Several investigators have looked at such a question and calculated the annual cost. Let us look at one conservative analysis (Health Aff (Millwood). 2010 Sep; 29(9): 1569–1577). The investigators added up the different direct and indirect costs of our medico-legal system from 2008. This is detailed in Table #25. First listed are the direct costs of how much money was awarded plaintiffs for damages ($5.72 billion) and the legal and administrative costs of pursing and defending the cases ($4.13 billion). They then added to this the much higher indirect costs. That includes the cost of defensive medicine that is practiced because of the pressures of the system ($45.59 billion) and lost physician time spend defending such cases ($0.2 billion). That totals to $55.6 billion per year or 2.4% of all our healthcare spending in this country. Remember, this is a very conservative estimate. Other researchers think it might be as high as 10% of all the money we spend on medical care. Think of where that money could have gone instead to keep us healthy. In 2007, the per capita spending on healthcare in the United States was $7,538. That meant if we had fixed our medical liability problem, then, changing nothing else, we could have insured over more 7 million Americans.

Table 25. Annual Direct and Indirect Costs of Medical Liability in the United States (2008)

Taken from Health Aff (Millwood). 2010 Sep; 29(9): 1569–1577

Component	Cost ($ Billions)
Direct	
Payments for economic damages	$3.15
Payment for non-economic damages	$2.40
Payment for punitive damages	$0.17
Total payments for damages	**$5.72**
Plaintiff legal expenses	$2.00
Defendant legal expenses	$1.09
Other legal system expenses	$3.04
Total legal system expenses	**$4.13**
Indirect	
Hospital defensive medicine costs	$38.79
Physician defensive medicine costs	$6.80
Total defensive medicine costs	**$45.59**
Lost clinician time	$0.20
Total	**$55.64 billion**

There are other costs from our broken malpractice system that cannot be measured in dollar and cents. Take medical records. We already have seen that the first master of what goes into today's medical records is the medical insurance industry. That is, the emphasis is not so much on providing accurate, concise medical information as it is trying to prove to the billers that work was done, by giving them the information, *they* want to see. Today's medical records have a second master, the liability system. The second emphasis in writing (keyboarding, since it is mostly EMRs) is to create the impression that the clinician did everything in the correct manner and the patient knew of all the possible risks and complications. That is why medical records often read like court documents or real estate papers from a house closing, rather than, um...medical records! Because of the defensive attitude inherent to such writing, often it is impossible to figure out what really happened in a particular case. It is not unlike your teenage daughter's account what happened with her fender bender car accident. Meaning, she was not lying, but she was not exactly telling the truth, either. Therefore, medical liability is yet another barrier to the dissemination of accurate medical information.

Finally, medical malpractice cases and the threat of them contribute to practitioner burnout. Although factors that separate physician from the patient, such as electronic medical records, are primary causes of undue stress on medical staff, lawsuits play a significant role, too. Studies have shown that physicians who have had a medical malpractice claim recently filed against them are more likely to have burnout symptoms that those who have not. We, doctors, take claims against them to heart. They are crushing blows to us. Both the selection process in picking future physicians and medical training instill in us a need for perfectionism. Not only are we never allowed to make a mistake, we must always have all the answers. We must do it all, ourselves. We are lone wolves, never allowed to show weakness or vulnerability. A lawsuit is a direct slap in our face to this thinking and creates cognitive dissonance. Even if we never had a malpractice suit filed against us, the threat of it is never far for our thoughts. No one can work, effectively, day in and day out with a loaded gun pointed at their head. This leads to burnout. Physician burnout, in turn, leads to depression and anxiety, a higher rate of drug abuse, alcoholism and suicide, personal and professional problems and early retirement. Ironically, it leads to a poorer medicine service product that we all receive.

Let us summarize what we have learned about the medical liability system in the United States, today. It does not meet its first criteria, compensating victims of medical errors. Most of the money generated by the system pays to keep the system going rather than going to injured patients. Those patients who do receive payments, more often than not, were not victims of medical malpractice. And most victims of such malpractice never receive a dime from the system. It does not meet its second criteria for its existence, to reduce medical errors. Medical errors are rampant in our hospitals and all throughout our healthcare system, despite the high cost of liability. Finally, our present system generates a lot of societal cost because of defensive medicine efforts and practitioner burnout. Both make medical care less safe and effective as it should be as well as more expensive.

Let us look at how our SPUN Healthcare Plan can fix our medical liability insurance system. Let us start by looking what malpractice reforms have been proposed over the years. The first type is placing checks and balances on our present system. These are, by far, the most common proposals on the table, today. That includes limits or caps on the dollar amount of certain components of malpractice awards. Such awards are divided into economic and non-economic. Economic awards reimburse the victim for out of pocket medical costs, lost wages and ongoing expenses for care because of the malpractice occurrence. Non-economic awards are for physical and emotional pain and suffering. They also include punitive damages which are punishments against the injuring party for their reckless conduct. Limits that are proposed and enacted in some states are on these non-economic malpractice awards.

Other proposals are restrictions on the functioning of the liability system. For example, they might limit the amount time after a malpractice event that a lawsuit can be filed. They may require certain expert testimony before a lawsuit can proceed. All these limits do slightly reduce the stress on medical providers and decrease the number of unfairly rewards plaintiffs. However, they would not solve the fundamental problems of the system of reducing poorly practiced medicine and compensated the injured victims. We must go much further than this Band-Aid fix with our malpractice reform proposals.

The second set of proposed liability reforms are creating a guidelines-based judgment system. Under such a medicolegal system, the defendant, whether it be a hospital, physician or other healthcare worker would be judged against a standard book of care rules for a particular diagnosis or medical situation. This would replace the often conflicting and complex testimony of expert witnesses. It would make what is considered the standard of care, truly a standard of care. Although a logical step in medical tort reform as it would reduce the number of patients receiving claims that do not deserve them, it does not address all the other issues. Patients who have had damages done to them still would not be compensated and the toxic atmosphere that liability creates in American medicine still would remain.

A similar proposal for reform is an enterprise system. With this proposal, the medical care system is the entity that is insured. It, in turn, insures all its workers, including physicians. This moves the burden of policing the quality of care from the medico-legal system to the enterprise system. For a physician who practices poor medicine will have more lawsuits and drive up the cost of insurance for the entire system. It gives such networks more power to monitor the care of its healthcare providers. With more and more physicians working for someone, whether it be a hospital, hospital system or physician network, enterprise malpractice is becoming a reality. It has the potential to improve the quality of patient care. However, it does not address the problem of compensating the right victims of malpractice.

A more radical proposal is replacing our entire legal system of malpractice with a binding arbitration one. If a patient thinks she has been harmed by a practitioner, she would submit her claim to a mediator. This is someone outside the legal system. The mediator would judge the case based on its merit after hearing evidence from both sides. Binding arbitration is much faster, less expensive and less bureaucratic than today's court system. It also is fairer as experts are making the final decisions on complex medical cases, rather than a lay jury. Many practitioners, already, use this system. Patients, when seeking care from such practitioners, sign an agreement to use binding arbitration rather than the legal system.

Such a system of binding arbitration has the potential to improve our present medico-legal system. It is less expensive, faster and fairer to all than what we have today. It has the potential to improve medical care because the feedback from such a system would be more in line with the actual quality of care than with our present tort legal system. Am I saying this is the way to go with our SPUN Healthcare System? No, for we can do even better!

Today's system worries too much about pointing the finger of blame at someone. That someone is a physician, healthcare worker, hospital or practice. More important is that if someone has injuries, they need care. Let our system provide such care. How? By giving them corrective medical care and compensating them for lost income. The medical care part will be easy under our SPUN system, since it already is fully covered. This is another example of the beauty, simplicity and logic of universal healthcare. The lost income part will be one of four forms, depending on the case. There will be partial or full temporary disability benefits while the patient is recovering. For example, if you fall out of bed while in the hospital and break your arm, you will get a percentage of your income until your fracture heals. It would not matter if it is the hospital's fault because they let a blood pressure cuff on the floor and you tripped over it or if you were just clumsy. The second form will be partial or full permanent disability for lost wages. Following this first example, let us say if you broke your arm while you are in the hospital and you were a starting pitcher for the Philadelphia Phillies (Things like this always seem to happen to my hometown baseball team in real life.) and could never pitch again, then you will get payments for the rest of your life. The third form will pay for your retraining to another profession. Following our example, the system will pay for you to retrained to be a first baseman or a baseball coach. Finally, there will a life insurance policy for your family if the injury caused your death. Therefore, if you fell out of the fifth-floor window at that hospital, then your spouse and children will collect on a life insurance policy from your injury. If this system sounds vaguely familiar to you, it should. It is how today's workman's compensation systems are set up. Or, it is like a no-fault medical insurance policy of your car insurance. Such an insurance pays to take care of your injuries after a car accident, regardless of who was at fault in causing the crash.

Who will pay for such insurance under SPUN? Following our model of workman's compensation or no-fault car insurance, it will be a private insurance company. Such an insurance company will write policies for anyone or any organization that is involved in healthcare in the United States. The insurance will be a requirement to practice under the SPUN system. The practitioners, whether they be dentists, physicians or hospitals, will pay the premiums. The premiums will be based on several factors, including the specialty and the rate of claims. High risk fields, like obstetrics will have higher premiums as will practitioners with more claims. Since all medical care already is covered under SPUN, the premiums only will have to cover the lost wages, retraining and death benefits of today's tort system. That means, regardless of specialty, the premiums will be significantly lower than today's malpractice premiums.

Who would decide if there was a healthcare related injury? Any potential case will be submitted to a member of a specific panel of experts employed by SPUN for such a purpose. They will review and decide all the cases presented to them by injured patients. Such experts will be physicians and other medical professionals experienced in the injury-related field. For example, if there was a question of a neurological injury from birth trauma, the case will be reviewed by a pediatric neurologist. A bone fracture will be reviewed by an orthopedic surgeon. If the patient was not happy with the decision, they could appeal to a higher tier appeal panel of the SPUN Healthcare Plan. Such a reviewer's task will be made much easier than it is today for medical malpractice cases. Why? All the records of the case in question will be standardized and centralized in the SPUN system of universal medical records.

The injured patient would have to prove just three things to the reviewer. First, their injury was the result of medical care. Second, their injury was preventable. And third, the treatment was not medically the correct action. Remember the reviewers are not assigning fault. Fault is not important if someone is hurt. Let us instead get the patient better, give them compensation for their lost time and wages and get them back as productive members of society. Since determining whether an injury occurred is a much easier task than determining if malpractice occurred, the review process will be much simpler. This will reduce the time and money spend on the legal processes to make that determination. This will put more money in the hands of the injured and less in the hands of the lawyers and the bureaucrats.

Also, all significantly injured patients will be covered. That would include relatively minor injuries not covered today because the legal expenses do not justify the filing of a medical malpractice case. There will be some commonsense criteria in reviewing a claim. There will be certain minimum thresholds for medical injuries. This will be defined by missing at least seven days of work, being partially or permanently disabled from the injury or have died from it. The patient will have a limited but reasonable time of three years after injury to file the claim. No lawyer will be needed. But if a lawyer was employed, it will be on a fee basis, not a percentage basis, like with today's tort system.

Think of the positive effects on healthcare from such a

liability system. There will be less coverup and more information given to a patient by practitioners when an injury occurs. That is because the concept of "fault" has been removed from the equation. Medical care providers will volunteer and inform patients and their families when medical injuries occur, so they can get the financial assistance they deserve.

Such a system will remove practitioners' fear of medical malpractice. There will of no sense of that evil, arbitrary Nazi prison guard looking over every healthcare worker's shoulder, every minute of every working day. Medicine will be practiced based on science and rationality. Medical practitioners from the chief of neurosurgery at Johns Hopkins to the newest hired hospital orderly there will feel empowered to do the right thing. Medical records will be simpler and more accurate in describing the medical facts of a case, not defensively written as they are today. Informed consent will be an educational process for the patient, not a complex and legalese one. Cesarean sections rates will fall across the nation. There will be so few CT scans and MRIs performed, we could send the unused diagnostic equipment to where they are truly needed in the Third World. The total cost of medical care will drop. Both dollar and cents terms and in the form of the fewer needless tests, surgeries, complications and pain. We all will be healthier for less money.

You may ask if such no-fault compensation systems exist, today? Yes, even in the United States! Florida and Virginia each have small, voluntary, pilot programs set up for compensating babies with neurological injuries at birth. Such injuries are a huge source of litigation today and this system is a solution that two states have found that works. Families can opt for such a program. When they do, they give up their rights for using the traditional tort system should a birth injury occur. Physicians and hospitals that are part of the plan pay into it an annual premium. Claims are presented to the Workers' Compensation Commission in Virginia and an administrative law judge from the State Management Department in Florida. If they decide a neurologic injury occurred, no fault is assigned. But the child receives payment for all future medical and related care and even future lost earnings. Studies of these programs have discovered they are financially sound. That obstetricians practice better and less defensive medicine and have lower total insurance premiums. Finally, and most important of all, injured children are better compensated than they would have been under a tort system.

Some countries have instituted such a system but cover all medical injuries. Sweden, Finland, New Zealand, Australia and the providence of Quebec in Canada have some form of non-fault medical injury compensation system. Let us explore Sweden's program which is cited as an ideal model of how such a system would work. Up until 1975, Sweden had a traditional tort system for medical malpractice claims. To cover more medically injured patients, the country converted to a no-fault system that was bundled with the country's workman compensation plan. The plan covers all medical care events that cause a physical injury. The injury must have been serious enough to result in at least a month of lost wages, permanent disability or death. There is a three-year time limit to file a claim. To have a valid claim, the Swedish patient must show there is a direct connection between a medical treatment and the injury, the treatment was not medically necessary, and the injury was avoidable. The compensation is standardized and is given to the patient as a percentage of wages lost. A Swedish insurance company, the PSR, makes the determination if the patient's claim is valid. A patient can appeal to two higher levels is he is not happy with the insurance company's decision. Unlike the proposed SPUN no-fault plan, a Swedish patient can go outside their system and sue in a traditional court if he wishes. The Swedish plan is financed through a combination of funds from the general tax fund, a tax on healthcare visits and premiums paid by the physicians and hospitals. The system is extremely efficient. Over 80% of the premiums go to patient claims compared to just 40% in the American malpractice system. Therefore, the premiums are very low for the practitioners. Unlike for our proposed SPUN plan, the premiums are not based on the claims made against them.

I hear those of you out there who feel any system from Sweden must smack with socialism and therefore, by definition, is not acceptable in the United States. But dear reader, we have such a similar system in our country, today. Though not part of healthcare directly, it is a system for paying for medical care. It is our no-fault car insurance plans. Such plans pay for medical injuries from automobile accidents, regardless of who caused the collision. It reduces the cost for the system by saving money litigating who was responsible. It cuts to the chase and takes care of the injured and does not bother with assigning blame. No-fault plans grew of the frustration of the rising car insurance premiums everyone was starting to pay, beginning in the 1960s. Future presidential candidate Michael Dukakis, while he was state senator in Massachusetts, was instrumental in passing the country's first no-fault car insurance plan in 1967. The plan spread to many other states, where it is either mandatory or the driver can pick either a no-fault or traditional tort system plan. (Of course, car insurance rates are lower with the no-fault plan where there is a choice!)

You may accept that our no-fault plan will compensate more patients that are injured undergoing treatment. You may accept that it is a fairer system. You may accept that it is a less expensive system to administrate. You even may accept that it will reduce the rate of defensive medicine practice. But you may argue how will it deter malpractice or the high instances of injury from medicine in the United States and make us healthier. The answer, it cannot. Although the rate of no-fault claims will affect a provider's insurance premium, it is not enough to weed out bad physicians and hospitals. What our healthcare system needs is a separate system from this proposed compensation model to evaluate its practitioners. We need a simple, fair and strong system to evaluate our well we are being taken care of.

How would our SPUN Healthcare Plan make sure those who take care of us do not harm us? When I was practicing medicine, I constantly was asked for recommendations for a top-notched physicians or other healthcare providers. For example, who is the best family physician, cardiologist, general surgeon, physical therapist or psychologist. Even today with me being retired from practice, a week does not go by that a friend or family member will not call me with such a question. (Except today, it usually is by text rather than by phone call.) Typically, my first response is a sarcastic one, "You do not want to know who the best physician is, you want to avoid the worst one." In my experience, most, 90% or more, of healthcare providers provide excellent medical care. If you pick any medical provider in that ninety percent, you will get the care you need without additional risk of injury. But you want to avoid that bottom ten percent. That way, physicians are no different than any other profession or career. Whether we are looking at lawyers, accountants, restaurants, plumbers or truck drivers, there is a normal distribution bell-shaped curve to their required skills and abilities.

The problem of the ten percent extends beyond the poor care they give. The ten percent can drag down the work of the usually competent and hard-working ninety percent. I think back to when we had a group of a dozen or so medical students on a rotation in our obstetric department. Sometimes there would be a truly superior student in the group. That student would put in extra hours, go out of the way to be helpful, was extra inquisitive and a pleasure to work with. An interesting effect took place. The usual middle of the road students, seeing this exceptional one, would step up their game a notch or two. Soon, the whole group was working at a superior level. The opposite of this effect would happen, too. There would be a student who was a slacker and did not put much effort in. He would show up late and leave early. You could read the disinterest in his face. Again, the usual middle of the road students, seeing him, would drop their work ethic, and the entire group was poor performing. That happens with working professionals, too, not just students. Seeing and working day in and day out with the bottom ten percent can be demoralizing. It can lead many professionals that normally would be in the middle of the competency pact to let up on their professional game. Incompetency, like the flu, is contagious.

How do we find that bottom ten percent? Today, physicians, other healthcare professionals, medical practices and hospitals are assessed in many and varying ways. Let us describe them, review how effective they are in finding the ten percent, and see which ones our SPUN Healthcare Plan should use. First, there are online survey websites such as health grades, Angie's List and Ratemds. They are no different than the user ratings that are available for restaurants like Open Table or for books at Amazon. There are not very scientific, as they express the opinions of just those patients web savvy enough and motivated enough to do such surveys. Certainly, by themselves, they are not the be all and end all for determining the competency of a practitioner. They do serve a purpose. They are helpful for potential patients in getting a flavor for the practice in terms of the friendliness of the staff, wait times in the office, responsiveness to phone calls and personality of the practitioner.

A slight improvement in medical provider evaluation is a scientifically performed one. They are performed by third-party opinion takers, hired for that purpose by health organizations. I am sure if you have gone to any hospital or hospital-related practice or system, you have not escaped a phone call, text, email or snail mail urging you to assess your encounter. Although part of the reason for self-assessment is to lead to self-improvement, to find where there are weak links in the delivery of care, there is a more cynical reason for such surveys. Money. Since the passage of the Affordable Care Act, hospital reimbursement rates for Medicare are tied to patient satisfaction scores. In addition, many private medical insurance companies tie their reimbursement rates for providers to how happy patients are with their medical care. Physicians employed by larger organizations, such as healthcare networks and hospitals, usually have their pay or bonus partially determined by their scores.

How valuable are such scientifically conducted survey scores? Satisfaction scores do help health organizations and physicians determine their strengths and more importantly, see their weaknesses, so they can focus on what needs improvement. For example, when I was working as a physician, the network I was employed by used the Press Ganey Associates to assess our practice. They found we had problems with our telephone system, patients getting appointments in a timely manner and wait times in the office. This was a created opportunity to improve our practice by focusing in on our deficiencies. Also, hospitals and medical practices with higher patient scores make more money and have lower rates of medical malpractice lawsuits than those with low scores. This is not unexpected. This is no different from restaurants with excellent Open Table ratings make more money than those with poor ones.

But patient satisfaction scores are to healthcare professionals what standardized student test scores are to school teachers. A metric to solve or try to work around rather than a true measure of performance. For teachers, it is to teach for the standardized test rather than impart true skill and knowledge. For healthcare workers, it means giving patients what they want rather than what they need. These often are entirely different things. For in medicine, sometimes you must make a patient unhappy to give him proper healthcare. For example, if an obese patient comes in for a routine health checkup, a physician may make that patient "happy" by avoiding a discussion of his weight, diet and exercise. But this obviously is poor medical practice. Patient satisfaction scores contributed mightily to today's opioid crisis in the United States. Starting in the early 1990s, patients were surveyed as to how well their pain was controlled when they were in a health facility as part of patient satisfaction scores. This led to physicians overprescribing narcotics to get a good score rather than challenging their medication abuse. Physicians often order expensive and sometimes dangerous medical tests and do unnecessary procedures on patients they know are useless for fear of a bad patient review. Hospitals spend money to create spa-like feel to their buildings and have gourmet meals served in their cafeteria rather than properly staffing their wards.

Our future healthcare system must balance between giving patients the right to review their medical providers and having these reviews adversely influence how practitioners practice medicine. The answer is simple. Take away the *direct* connection between patient satisfaction scores and financial incentives. Of course, we will continue to allow outside organizations conduct surveys on health practitioners and organizations. Of course, if organizations and practices want to do their own surveys to find their weakness and strengths, they should be permitted. The SPUN Healthcare System, as part of its system of universal medical records, will have its own assessment system. Here patients can give reviews and fill out questionnaires about the care they reviewed. This will create a nationwide, searchable database for everyone to help locate the best fit of practitioner for them. But by untying pay and reimbursement from such survey results, it will take away the incentive to cheat the system. Physicians, other healthcare workers, hospitals and other medical organizations then can concentrate to delivering the right care rather than winning a popularity contest.

Licensing is the next method of assessing health professionals and organizations for their competency. Let us review how licensing works for American physicians, nurses and hospitals as representative of the major types of providers. The individual states do the professional licensing process. For example, there is no single national physician medical license. In my home state, Pennsylvania, medical licensing is just one of dozens of controlled professions that includes an odd mixture of careers including engineers, geologists, accountants, real estate agents and barbers. States vary as to what careers require licenses, but every state requires their physicians to have a license to practice.

The medical license requirements vary from state to state. All require a physician graduate from an accredited American medical school. Foreign medical school graduates also can be licensed. But they typically have a tougher road by having to jump through more hoops to get their license. (Sorry for mixing my metaphors.) The physician then must pass one of several different licensing examinations and have a number of years of residency training after medical school graduation. The other varying requirements include letters of recommendation, background checks, fingerprinting, interviews and medical malpractice insurance. The medical license is only for practicing medicine in a single state. That makes it tricky if a physician moves out of state or is locum tenens (a physician who fills in temporary in a healthcare position and travels from position to position all around the country). With the technologic advance of practicing medicine online, this practice of medicine across state lines has become more complicated.

Medical licenses are renewed periodically. In Pennsylvania, for example, this happens every even-numbered year. During the renewal process, the physician's credentials are reviewed. To maintain a license, each state requires certain activities. In Pennsylvania, that includes maintaining malpractice insurance and having a certain amount and type of continuing medical education.

Physician relicensing seems like an ideal time to periodically assess the competency of practicing physicians. However, only obvious and serious issues of competency are questioned. These include drug or alcohol abuse and impairment, losing hospital privileges and criminal conduct. Interestingly, they ask about malpractice suits which as we have seen are not predictive of physician competency. Certainly, these are serious matters that deserve attention when it is the time to renew a physician's license. But they do not go far enough. They do not answer the very basic question of whether the physician knows what she is doing.

The requirements for a nursing license are similar to a medical license. To become a nurse requires a formal education. There are two trends in nursing education, today. More registered nurses and more nurses with bachelor's degrees. At the most basic, there are two basic types of nurses: licensed practice nurses and (LPN) and registered nurses (RN). LPNs perform more basic nursing care and have less years of education compared to RNs. Although the demand for both is growing, there is more demand for the more skilled RN. There are three educational pathways to become an RN: diploma, associate and bachelor. A diploma program is mostly practical, hospital-based learning. An associate program combines some classroom and theory to the nursing education. The college-based bachelor program has even more concept and theory learning. Today's trend is toward the requirement of a bachelor's degree for all registered nurses. This reflects the increasing complexity of today's medicine. The second requirement for a nursing license is passing a written test, the National Council Licensure Examination (or NCLEX-RN for short).

Like physicians, nurses must renew their professional licenses. Like physicians, nursing licenses are issued at the state level and the requirements vary. In Pennsylvania, nurses renew their licenses every two years. To do so, they must do a certain number of hours of continuing education but only answer questions about serious impairment activities like crimes and drug abuse. Again, like physicians, nurses do not have to prove they know what they are doing. It is true that one can maintain a nursing license without really knowing how to take a blood pressure.

The process for licensing hospitals and other medical facilities is only a bit more complex. Again, it is done at the state level with each state having different requirements. Hospitals, to obtain and maintain their license to operate, have to offer in-patient healthcare services and maintain certain facilities like a clinical laboratory, diagnostic x-ray services and a surgical suite. As we shall see, like for the physician and the nurse, the major regulation of hospitals does not happen at the level of the license. Think of licensing in medicine like licensing to drive a car. You only need a certain minimal driving skill to get a driver's license and you need to show that minimal skill, only once. It is renewed periodically without difficulty, as long as the driver has not gotten into too much trouble with his driving since the previous renewal. But just like driver licensing is no guarantee of the quality of your driving, medical licensing is no guarantee of the safety of the medical provider.

Our present medical tort system does not work. Patient satisfaction surveys do not work. Licensing does not work. Even our proposed SPUN compensation system will not work. We still have not answered the question how healthcare quality is assured or should be assured in this country. Today, the answer is credentialing. Credentialing is an organization's process to make sure a healthcare provider had the adequate training and remains qualified to provide healthcare. Do you remember the Leonardo DiCaprio movie "Catch Me If You Can"? The film is based on the real-life story of Frank Abagnale who was a con artist who posed as many professionals from airline pilot to criminal prosecutor. One of his cons was as a Georgia physician. Credentialing stops a potential Frank Abagnale from practicing medicine.

How does today's credentialing process work? Let us start with the process for credentialing physicians. All physicians must go through the process when they apply to work at a new healthcare facility or when they apply to part of a health insurance network. Examples of the first type of credentialing process include a surgeon applying to operate a particular outpatient surgical center, an obstetrician wanting to deliver babies at a certain hospital or if an emergency care physician starting work at a new urgent care center. The second type occurs if a physician wants to be paid the going rate by a medical insurance company. A physician must go through a credentialing process for every insurance company of every one of his patients.

Right off the bat you can see a problem created by credentialing. A physician might be working at four different hospitals, two different outpatient centers and have patients with ten different health insurance plans. That physician would have to go through 16 different credentialing processes. It becomes perpetual motion. If you are a physician, at some time, someone wants to renew and review your credentials. A second problem is that each entity has its own standards of credentialing. You can image it must be harder to get your credentials at Johns Hopkins University Hospital in Baltimore or the Cleveland Clinic than it is to get credentials at Nowhereville County Clinic.

The actual physician credentialing process is a more involved investigation than what is required for just a medical license. The investigation of a potential credentialed physician's background, education, malpractice, references is similar. But credentialing goes much further. It looks into a physician's postgraduate training for a specialty or subspecialty. Virtually all physicians specialize in a particular field of medicine. There are no true "general practitioners" anymore for even family medicine is its own specialty. To be a specialist, a physician must complete a residency training of three to seven years after medical school and pass a series of oral and written tests unique to the specialty. Specialists must maintain their standards by required continuing education and periodic retesting. Subspecialists are specialist's specialists. For example, cardiology is a subspecialty of internal medicine, neonatology is a subspecialty of pediatrics and infertility is a subspecialty of obstetrics and gynecology. Subspecialists must complete what is called a fellowship training of one to three years after residency and pass their own set of tests and maintain their own required continuing education and periodic retesting. For although theoretically with a just a medical license, an allergist would be allowed to do a heart transplant surgery, credentialing, at the level of the hospital and the medical insurance payer, prevents that from happening. At the hospital level, what practitioners can and cannot do are called their privileges. For example, when I was practicing obstetrics and gynecology, I had hospital privileges to deliver babies and perform hysterectomies but not to do heart bypass surgery (Thank goodness.).

So, who ensures that specialists and subspecialists have these "specialized" medical skills? Not the state licensing board or similar state or federal agency. Instead, it is determined by various non-profit organizations called "boards." To fully understand specialty boards, I will tell you a tale of why the mere mention of the city of Chicago gives me cold chills down my spine after an experience that happened more than thirty years ago. After I finished my four-year residency in obstetrics and gynecology, like all graduating residents, I took a written multiple-choice test to demonstrate that I knew enough about the specialty to practice on my own. The test was given by the American Board of Obstetrics and Gynecology. Founded in 1927, it is the sole arbitrator of who is and isn't a specialist in the field for the United States. But completing a residency training and a passing a written test are not enough. During my second year in private practice, I had to collect my "cases." Basically, it is all the information about the patients I took care of during that year. Collecting cases is a monumental task. Obstetrician-gynecologist will see thousands of different patients during one year of practice. My case list then was submitted to the board to ensure that my practice of the specialty had enough breadth and depth. Meaning, I saw enough patients with enough variety of problems typically seen in the field. Once my case list was accepted, I then could take the oral examinations, the final step of becoming a full-fledged or "board-certified" obstetrician-gynecologist.

Professional examinations have a legendary aura attached to them for their associated pain and torture. I am sure you have heard tales of horror about the Certified Public Accountant test or the bar examination for lawyers. Although not as well known, the oral examination for the medical specialties has a similar reputation. For months ahead of time, I studied for this test while still working full time, taking shifts of 24 hours of on call and raising a young family. I took a week-long review course that met from 8 am to 8 pm, each day. (Of course, this expensive course was given by the same physicians who administered the test! Talk about conflict of interest!) Finally, I paid a four-digit fee for the honor of taking the test and had to fly to windy and cold Chicago in December to take it. (The test has since moved to the much warmer city of Dallas.)

When I arrived in Chicago, I discovered that ABOG took over a hotel across the street from the Willis (then Sears) Tower. I do not think it was a good idea having such a tall building so close to a group of suicidal examinees. Entering the hotel, I came upon a scene from the Zombie Apocalypse. For it was full of bleary-eyed, jet-lagged, unspeaking men and women awaiting their fate. Everyone was dressed in the same style business suit, not daring to stand out in the crowd. No one spoke to or acknowledged their fellow zombie. The evening before the test, the hotel restaurant was full of them dining at tables for one. The zombies were eating their last meal of Chicago steak while simultaneously cramming facts from opened notebooks and textbooks stacked in front of them.

The oral examination process went on for a full week. Each examinee was scheduled for either a morning or afternoon test on a particular day. I had the misfortune of having an afternoon test. That meant I had to watch the results of the morning gladiators versus lions' battles. It was not pretty. For the lions were well fed that day. The stories of the horrors of the morning tests spread among us. One of the examinees had to be sent by ambulance to the hospital as he developed chest pain during his oral test. We zombies in the hotel did have a strange empathy for him. We were more worried that he would have to come back in a year to face his uncompleted oral examinations again than the condition of his coronary arteries.

When the time for my testing came, I reported to one of the small courtesy rooms at the hotel. A group of a dozen of us received our instructions from a "good Nazi." We were informed how the examination horror stories were mere exaggerations. That the examinations, instead, will be a fun, intellectual challenge for us. Like appearing on the game show, Jeopardy. That we would enjoy our encounter with each of the three oral examiners that we would meet that afternoon. Finally, we all were wished a "safe trip, home."

Oddly, the actual examinations took place in the hotel's guests' bedrooms. Feeling a bit more at ease, I knocked on the hotel room door of my first examiner. Upon entering, I saw a bizarre scene that could have been painted by Salvador Dali. It was a typical businessperson's hotel room with a queen-sized bed, bureau and television. Sitting in a chair at the foot of the bed was a casually attired middle-aged man. I felt so overdressed in my zombie suit, like I wrongly interpreted the dress instructions on a wedding invitation. His feet were propped up on the bed. His hands cradled his head. He looked like he was sunning at the beach. He did not make a move to greet me as if I was a member of the hotel staff. In front of him, on the bed, was a small carousel of slides, a projector and screen (The twentieth century equivalent of a Power Point presentation for those of you too young to know.) As I walked into the room, he tossed me, without a warning, the remote for the projector. Was catching fly balls was a qualification for my specialty? As I scooped up the remote control, he pointed to the empty chair next to him. He ordered me to "Sit down, doctor!" By his tone and body language, he had turned this personal address of respect and education to one of distain and sarcasm. He was saying "You think you are a doctor? For the next hour, I will prove you wrong." There was no modest attempt at pleasantries. No chit-chat. There was no introduction or exchange of names. Why would he risk the possibility of the Stockholm Syndrome kicking in?

I sat down uncomfortably close to him. I felt him invading my personal space. He ordered me to click my remote control to the first slide. It was a picture of a non-stress test. This is the most basic test performed in obstetrics. It is test that an intern on the first day of work can understand and interpret. It was a hanging curve ball of a question, setting me up for the hundred mile per mile fastballs to come. The examiner, still in his sunning on his beach posture, asked me if I knew what was shown on the screen. I answered, "non-stress test." I hesitated, at first, sensing a trap. He responded with a long "Ohhhhhh!!!" He seemed surprised that I got this simple question correct. The he asked a second question. He asked if I used non-stress tests in my practice. Again, he addressed me as "doctor," his voice full of sarcasm. I answered "yes." With my words barely off my lips, he sat up suddenly in his chair and fired back at me

"When?" I answered with a long laundry list of obstetric indications for using a non-stress test. Halfway through my list, as I was listing a pregnant woman past her due date, he interrupted me, again. "Postdates.... ahhhh!" "So, doctor, how long will you let a pregnant woman go past her due date before you will induce labor?" With a huge lump in my throat, I answered "Depends..." Again, he jumped in, "Depends on what?" I answered with another laundry list of variables that would affect my decision. I stated it would include the condition of the pregnant woman's cervix. With a rapid-fire response, he asked "What if the cervix was like this?" As he spoke, he pounded the side table next to him with his clenched fist. He was indicating that the cervix was firm and not ready to be in labor. But he looked like Khrushchev with his shoe at the United Nations.

The rest of his inquisition followed this intimidating script. A barrage of questions alternating with interruptions. The distaining use of the "doctor" address. Answers I knew were interrupted before I could finish. Answers I did not know were pursued with predator efficiency. He was sarcastic, one minute. Patronizing, the next. A blur of slide pictures flew by on the screen. I never felt so overwhelmed, incompetent or stupid, any other time in my life. Finally, when my oral examination time was up, he led me to my next examiner. He ended with the scripted "Have a safe trip, home." The rest of that afternoon with other two examiners were no better. These encounters were such a blur, all I remember today were the endings with the "Have a safe trip, home" line. I felt like I was that student that somehow slipped through the cracks of the system. Now, I was being discovered for the fraud I was. My final memory of that day was of a hotel courtesy van to back to the airport. It was full of us unspeaking zombies in our matching suits.

Somehow, I passed my oral examination. Up until 1986, that would have been it. I would have been considered board-certified for life. Unfortunately, I was born a little too late and passed the examination two years later in 1988. That meant, that I had to take a written examination to maintain that status, every ten years. Then, the rules changed yet again. There were written examinations are every six years. Then, the rules changed for a third time. ABOG required an additional step to maintain my certification. I had to read a minimum of 30 articles from the medical literature each year and take a test on each of them.

The cost for all these tests runs hundreds of dollars, annually. Because they are the only game in town, ABOG can charge what it wants and add on as many requirements as it wishes. All the other specialty boards work in the same way. They are monopolies. The boards make money giving the tests and the members of the board make money prepping the examinees to take the test. But all this expensive, time-consuming and at times, cruel testing do not assure the public that they are being taken care of by competent specialists. There must be a better way.

Let us get back to physician credentialing. It is not a one and done process. Credentialing is reassessed periodically. In addition, if a new procedure comes along, the physician must undergo a certain amount of prescribed new training in that procedure before she can do that procedure. When robotic surgery was introduced as a mainstream therapy, surgeons who wish to do such surgery had to undergo a certain amount of training in robotics and do a certain number of robotic surgeries under direct supervision before obtaining privileges for the technique.

Related to credentialing is the review process of physicians' competency by their hospital department. If a physician makes a major medical error or is found to have a weakness in a certain clinical situation, it is up to the department chairman of her specialty both to discover and to rectify it. For example, if a certain surgeon's patients are having a high rate of wound infection, the chairman of the department of surgery will be responsible both for finding out that the abnormal rate of infections are occurring and then review her surgical technique to see why it is occurring.

One process, hospital departments use to discover clinicians' problems is the century old tradition of American medicine called the Morbidity and Mortality Conference or "M and M" for short. As the "morbid" and "mortal" names imply, such conferences look at the causes of patient deaths and complications in each hospital department. Typically held monthly, they investigate why they happened and if they were preventable. The goal for M and Ms is to identify weaknesses in a department and fix them. M and Ms are peer reviewed, meaning doctors criticize themselves. The hope is that will lead to open and frank discussion among practitioners. To promote such openness, the proceedings from such gatherings are confidential and legally protected from disclosure at malpractice lawsuits.

We have seen a common theme in American medicine, today, what is good in theory fails in reality. For the effectiveness of M and Ms conferences is uneven. It is a lot to ask a group of physicians who know each other well and work with each other daily to criticized each other, even in a protected environment. Therefore, M and Ms can be times for coverups of incompetence or times for political vendettas within a hospital's department.

An example of the latter is what happened to a psychiatrist colleague and friend of mine, Larry. He was in practice for decades at the same hospital. Larry had earned a reputation of being a respected, hardworking and highly competent therapist. At one peer review meeting, he was viciously attacked for prescribing a medication "off label." This is the common and accepted practice of giving a medication to a patient for an indication that has not been approved by the Food and Drug

Administration. There was no complication from his off-label use of the medication. In fact, it was a clever and effective treatment for patients having severe anxiety while being on a ventilator while critically ill in the intensive care unit. The attack was not really about his competency but rather an attempt to force him off staff because of his age. Even though he was 80 years old at the time, he was up to date, sharp, witty and as intelligent as any other physician on staff, or maybe more so. But sadly, the thinly-veiled political attack worked, and Larry left the medical staff at that hospital.

Although some hospital departments and medical insurers do measure certain parameters of physician competence on a periodic basis, there is no set standards for such assessments. They vary widely from institution to institution and from insurance company to insurance company. Although credentialing remains the major means of assessing a physician's initial and on-going competence in the United States, it lacks established standards and objectivity, especially when looking at the established practitioner.

Let us turn our attention to nurses and their credentialing process. Modern nursing has evolved into a profession of hundreds of different specialized medical careers. When one thinks of a nurse, one stereotypes the profession by imaging the hospital nurse on a medical surgical floor. But the nurse anesthetist, who administers anesthesia in the operating room, the nurse practitioner, who is a mid-level medical care provider in the office or hospital, the nurse supervisor, who administrates departments of hundreds of workers, the public health nurse, who tracks down the cause and spread of disease in a community and the wound care nurse who specializes in the management of wound infections and other complications are just a few examples of this professional diversity. To become specialized in nursing, one must have a higher level of education, take more tests and maintain a more in-depth level of continuing education.

This education comes in the form of credentials and certifications. Credentials are like other advanced degrees that non-medical personnel earn. For example, such credentials include: master's degree for a nurse practitioner or an MBA for management position. Certifications show a more informal possession of specialized knowledge such as a possession of a certification in lactation consultation or nursing oncology.

Nursing assessment is not unlike that for workers in private industry. For virtually all nurses work for someone else, be it a hospital, clinic or private office practice. Nurses are assessed by their supervisors. That supervisor could be a nurse manager, office manager or physician employer. Bosses have their own standards. How fairly and how well a nurse is evaluated varies significantly from one place of employment to another. What is true of nurses is true of radiology technicians, occupational therapists, laboratory technologists and the other hundred specialized healthcare workers. We see there is not a consistent system of assessing the skills and knowledge of medical personnel on a continuous and fair basis to find the ten percent that are not competent.

Hospitals and other health facilities must maintain their accreditation, too. Part of the reason is to reassure the public that they are delivering safe medical care. But there is a more cynical reason. I have a friend who says the answer to nine out of ten questions in life is "money." Certainly, this is the real purpose of hospital accreditation. For without it, hospitals cannot be paid by governmental insurances like Medicare and Medicaid. The process of hospital accreditation is performed by independent non-profit assessment organizations. There are more than a dozen different ones in the United States. To make things even more complicated, hospitals can opt to have their accreditation process by the Centers for Medicare and Medicaid Services (CMS), which is a part federal, part state agency that administers government medical insurance.

By far the biggest hospital accreditation service is the Joint Commission, which surveys over 21,000 American hospitals. The Joint Commission inspects hospitals in a three-year cycle on hundreds of areas of operation. Until 2006, the timing of these inspections were known to the hospital. Like a platoon knowing when the drill sergeant will be checking the barracks, the days leading up to these inspections created a manic atmosphere in hospitals. Floors were vigorously scrubbed and waxed. Stretchers and IV poles that usually littered the hallways disappeared from view. Staff was drilled on vague hospital mission statements. Today, the Joint Commission's surveys are unannounced. Believe it or not, hospitals still drill for such visits by having mock surveys, like they do for large scale disaster planning.

To paraphrase Shakespeare, a hospital's Joint Commission accreditation is "full of sound and fury, signifying nothing." The Washington Post, in 2007, found that 99% of inspected hospitals get accredited. (Gaul, Gilbert M. Accreditors blamed for overlooking problems. The Washington Post. Pp. A01. 2007-07-17) The Joint Commission is supported by the hospitals it inspects and its board is full of hospital bigwigs. Therefore, it has a conflict of interest, by definition. For hospital accreditation, despite the expense of over $40,000 per hospital per evaluation and despite the all the work on both the hospital and the evaluators' ends, has not been shown to make for safer patient care. This is the conclusion of a complete review of all the studies in the medical literature looking at the impact of hospital accreditation on effective healthcare. (Brubakk, K., Vist, G. E., Bukholm, G., Barach, P., Tjomsland, O. A systematic review of hospital accreditation: the challenges of measuring complex intervention effects. BMC Health Services Research 2015 15:280.) Plus, all the resources spend by hospitals preparing for and fixing deficiencies after the accreditation processes are resources that could have been used to improve patient care, directly. Hospitals also have the challenge of meeting hundreds of other accreditation processes, big and small. Local, state and the federal governments, medical insurance companies and other independent medical care organizations continually are evaluating them, often with conflicting goals.

Some accreditation demands do patients more harm than good. For example, during the 1990s, the Joint Commission emphasized the assessment of pain that patients were experiencing while in the hospital and aggressively encouraged its treatment. Pain scores became known as the "fifth vital sign" (after pulse, temperature, respiratory rate and blood pressure). I am sure you all have been asked by a health professional when you go in for almost any type of encounter what you pain score is, from 0 to 10. Headache. Axe through skull. Routine physical. Blood pressure evaluation. It does not matter. On the surface, it seems reasonable to be concerned about patients' pain. However, this created a medical practice environment where there was an obsession with such scores and to lower the pain scores at all costs. All of us who worked in hospitals at that time heard how if we didn't address patients' pain scores, the Joint Commission would take away our hospital's accreditation. You know what happened next. The prescribing of narcotics exploded and now we are in the midst of an opioid addiction crisis. This is in part because of a well-intended but road to perdition regulation.

It is ironic that modern medicine which preaches evidence-based approaches, evaluates itself by processes that are not evidence-based. To summarize, the American healthcare system, today, has a multitiered structure to the licensing, evaluation and accrediting of its physicians, other healthcare workers, hospitals and other medical facilities. Like everything else of the system, it is complex, redundant and ineffective in its major task of identifying the ten percent of poor performing workers and institutions. It relies on an odd mixture of malpractice claims, patient generated reviews, state licensing and relicensing requirements, employer-based reviews, medical insurance company reviews and peer reviews. None of these do what they are supposed to do, improve the medical care we get. There must be a better way.

Let us take a wrecking ball to this expensive and ineffective provider evaluation system and build a new one from the ground up. To do so, we must list what characteristics such a healthcare evaluation system should possess. First, it must be simple. There should be one-stop shopping for licensing, relicensing, credentialing, recredentialing and identifying poor performing healthcare providers. It should be the same system for a physician, nurse, other healthcare worker or the hospital or facility, itself. Having one and only one evaluation mechanism lowers costs and reduces bureaucracy. Also, when medical deficiencies arise, it is hard to know in the beginning if the problem lies with the physician, hospital or elsewhere. Centralizing the system will solve this problem. Finally, everyone, everywhere in the country will be playing by the same rulebook of healthcare standards.

Second, the evaluation should be impartial. Physicians should not have the pressure of being the detective, prosecutor and judge of one's peers, as it is today. A nurse's career fate should not rest on the judgment of one manager. A hospital should not be audited by an organization that it is paying to support.

Third, the system should be constructive, not destructive. The goal is to fix the care deficiency, not close a hospital or put physicians and nurses out of work. I may be naïve, but I believe every healthcare worker and facility wants to provide good patient care, even those that are members of the ten percent. Too much is invested in them by our society's resources just to throw them all away. Once the ten percent are identified, just as much effort should be placed into rehabilitation as identification. Physicians and nurses can be retrained. Hospitals can change their systems of operation.

Fourth, the evaluation system should be transparent. Patients are consumers of health services. They deserve to know all that is known about their providers of services. It should be just like a car buyer, today, finding objective and open evaluation about an automobile's safety, like its crash testing results.

Finally, the evaluation system should look at everything. By focusing on just a few aspects of care, providers will focus on the test than on the total care. Plus, as we have seen, we do not know exactly what we should be evaluating to find the worrisome ten percent. So, until we do, let us look at everything.

Now let us build our medical provider evaluation system, together. As you guess, it is going to be run by the SPUN Healthcare Program, our national health insurance program. For the simple reason, if you control the purse strings of an operation, you control the entire operation. Since SPUN will be paying for virtually all American healthcare by controlling who will be paid, it is the obvious choice.

What will this national insurance system evaluation and credentialing system look like? SPUN will be responsible for licensing all healthcare workers and institutions in the country. Although we have been talking just about doctors, nurses and hospitals, the discussion is meant to use them as common illustrations of the entire industry. The national health plan will license dentists, physical therapists, radiology technicians, medical assistants, operating room scrub technicians, chiropractors and acupuncturists, just to name a few. It will issue licenses to same-day out-patient operating facilities, urgent care centers, extended care nursing homes and pharmacies as well as hospitals. This licensing will be a requirement, both to practice medicine in the United States and receive payment. SPUN licensing will replace everything else. Gone will be the state medical licensing boards, medical specialty credentialing, private insurance credentialing, hospital credentialing and the dozen other organizations that certify medical workers and institutions. SPUN not only control the first dimension of depth, reviewing all workers and facilities, the second dimension of width, replacing both licensing and credentialing, it will control the third dimension of length, reviewing providers from the first day of practice to the last.

Think how efficient such a system would be! Physicians could change jobs and move across the country without having to get a new state license with each move. Healthcare facilities would have access to any potential employee's work records in an instant (after getting the applicant's permission), streamlining hiring of all healthcare workers from a physical therapist to radiologist. There would be just one set of rules for everyone to follow covering everything from continuing education to fire safety.

SPUN will be objective in its review of healthcare. Local politics, friendships, personal prejudices and financial incentives will not influence competency. Sometimes being a bit detached from a situation is a good thing. SPUN, being completely independent, will make the best impartial decisions.

The SPUN's evaluation records will be available to anyone and everyone interested in the information. The records will be part of the SPUN medical app and website. From here, hospitals can view the credentials of a possible future employee. Patients can find the information about a potential physician they wish to use or hospital they might want to go to for care. Hospital surgical departments can compare their infection and other complication rates to their peers, anywhere in the country.

SPUN's primary goal in reviewing, licensing and credentialing healthcare will be to improve it, make it more efficient, effective and safer. All providers, from the part time medical assistant to the Chef of Surgery at the Mayo Clinic, from the tiniest rural pharmacy to Johns Hopkins Hospital, will receive a rating. As you know by now, I am obsessed with the lights of a traffic signal, so the overall rating will be summarized as green, red and yellow signals. Green light, meaning no problems, the provider, to paraphrase one of my old medical school professors, can "keep on, keeping on." They can continue practice medicine as they been, knowing they are providing excellent care. Red light means stop. It indicates a problem, so serious the provider should immediately stop providing care. The stoppage could be temporary or permanent, partial or complete. A surgeon may temporarily lose her license after a serious hand injury, until she can demonstrate it has healed. Obviously serious offenses like sexual misconduct, substance abuse, fraud and mis-prescribing of controlled medications will mean a permanent loss of license. A hospital that has serious problems in its labor and delivery suite may lose its obstetric license to practice, but if the rest of the facility has no significant problems, it can remain open. A nurse diagnosed with dementia, however, would have a complete suspension of his license.

The number of red lights will be relatively few. Just as important is finding practitioners who demonstrate an inadequacy of providing care that can be corrected but have not reached the point that they have lost their ability to provide care. These are the "ten percent" that we have been talking about this entire chapter. They will receive a yellow light. A surgeon performing cholecystectomies (removing diseased gallbladders) may have an abnormally high rate of infections, afterward. An obstetrician may have an unusually high cesarean section rate for his patients. A nurse may have difficulty taking a blood pressure "by hand," that is, without the aid of an automatic blood pressure cuff. Don't laugh, I knew an excellent nurse who gave great care, but her blood pressure readings were notoriously inaccurate. Many of us struggle with certain tasks with our professional performance, but otherwise are good healthcare providers. For example, I knew a gynecologist, who was an excellent practitioner, great surgeon and eventually went on to be a chief of a hospital's department. But he struggled his whole career making the correct diagnosis in cases of vaginal infections. Think what a blessing to his patients and to him if this problem was identified and he received some tailored education. All these yellow light practitioners need is some education and follow up evaluation. Both will be performed in a constructive, positive manner. The results of identifying and helping the yellow light "ten percent" will be better medical care for everyone. Not only will we be healthier, the system will save money by increasing the chance that the correct remedy is provided the first time.

What data will be collected to make these healthcare provider evaluations? In a word, everything. As we have seen, we are no yet sure what parameters truly matter to get us the best care. Also, the more data we collected, the less likely it will be that practitioners will try to game the system by concentrating on them and not all aspects of their care. Practically, this will start with all the information that the various healthcare evaluators collect already. It will include claims made to patients on behave of the no-fault malpractice system. It will include patient evaluations of practitioners and facilities. It will include all the initial and ongoing education that practitioners must and should do. But it must go further. It must include a complaint and reporting system for patients that they perceive is inadequate, dangerous, inappropriate or negligent. Along these lines, it also must include a peer complaint "whistle blower" reporting system where anyone in the field can report dangerous medical practices. Today, too much bad medical practices occur and then are ignored because of the fear of reprisal. Mistakes, bad practices and system failures are swept under the carpet, and workers look the other way out of fear of job loss. This is a serious lacking for there is a lot more than a defective service that is at stake. It is the everyone's life.

There will be a ton (or a terabyte?) of data to be mined from our centralized medical records. Here, one can find the breadth and depth of practice. Meaning is the practitioner doing enough of a certain procedure to remain sharp at it. For example, is a hospital performing enough open-heart surgeries? Is a surgeon doing enough robotic procedures to be adept? For medicine, as in the rest of human endeavors, you must continually use it or lose it. The SPUN EMR will generate reports on percentages of correct diagnoses, cure rates and complication rates. This will be performed for the top twenty conditions in each practitioner's field of specialty.

How will happen to all this mined data? It will be fed into reports tailored for each practitioner and be continuously updated. A dentist, nurse, general surgeon and radiologist each will have a unique type of report created. Hospitals, long-term nursing facilities and pharmacies will have their specific review, too. Reports without any problems will be published as green lights. Reports with a significant problem will create an alert at SPUN for immediate review. Reports with more minor issues also will be reviewed by SPUN on a less urgent basis. SPUN's independent reviewers will be practitioners of that specialty. Cardiologists will review cardiologists. Nurses will review nurses. Physical therapists will review physical therapists. The reviewers will decide if the information is serious enough to warrant either corrective action or even a suspension of part or all of one's delivering care. The goal is better patient care and every effort will be made to make as constructive as possible.

For we deserve better medical care that we are receiving today in the United States. The rate of preventable complications, system failures of health organizations and wasted allocations of resources is totally unacceptable. It costs us money and more importantly, cost us our lives. Today's review systems are too decentralized, not objective enough and not encompassing enough to identify these deficiencies. This problem is complicated by a medical legal tort system that punishes and rewards the wrong players. Its uneven justice has created a climate of fear among practitioners that ironically leads to even less effective and more expensive medical practices because of defensive medicine. We can do and must do better.

9. KEEP IT SIMPLE, SILLY

Now that I am retired, there are many things that I miss from my days of practicing obstetrics and gynecology. What I miss most is my patients. My field gave me the opportunity to develop relationships that were more than professional. I witnessed a woman's journey through her life. Usually starting with her as a college student, I watch her fall in love, make wedding plans and plan for a family. Then I guided her through her first pregnancy, labor and delivery. I saw her again for her second, third, fourth or sometimes even later pregnancy. We grew old together as our relationship lengthened. We noticed each other's extra gray hair at the time of her annual examination. We catch up on our careers, spouses and children. Although some obstetricians claim they get blamed if a baby they deliver grows up and fails AP Physics in high school, I found the exact opposite to be true. Women gave me undue credit for how wonderful their children turned out that I had the honor of delivering. For my response in such cases was always the same. "You do not thank the FedEx delivery person if an online order you placed turned out terrific."

It was a privilege to help women through many of life's tragedies. For as much happiness as obstetrics and gynecology can generate, its seemingly bipolar nature means it creates just as much pain, grief and sorrow. Infertility. Miscarriage. Stillborn. Birth defects. Newborn death. Cancer. It was a piece of cake to take of a patient when things were going so grand. For a health practitioner shows her abilities when things fall apart. The opportunity to make a tiny positive difference at these times is something I truly do miss.

You may be surprised to hear that the patient-doctor relationship as much receiving as it is giving. I cannot count the number of funny, sensitive, intelligent, talented, unique and resilient women I met in my career. Some had a sense of humor that could make me cry with laughter on days I was crying inside with sorrow. Some brought lunch to me during office hours, knowing I have not had the time to eat that day. Some wrote notes of appreciation that touched my soul. Some hugged me like a lost friend when meeting me on a random encounter at a grocery store. Some had fascinating tales of lives, events and careers that they shared with me and that I will never forget. Some inspired me with their grit through advanced cancer therapy, years of relentless infertility or months of prison-like, tortuous restrictions on a high-risk predelivery maternity hospital unit. Some trusted me, not only with their own care and lives, but the care and lives of their sisters, daughters, mothers and best friends. When I first wife was dying of cancer, they stepped in like they were my sisters. They gave when I needed it, without being asked.

Second, I miss witnessing the miracle of birth. It was a rare privilege. For I was able to participate in a living process that most people would just like to witness. For the beginnings and the ends of human lives are painful, messy, powerful and complicated. I guess they are like all the time in between. To see this incredible beginning of a new story, unfold, every day, was an honor.

I feel the same way about surgery. I miss that, too. It was

awe inspiring. Most laypeople think of surgery as repulsive or "yucky." But to see inside the body is to peer inside the workings of the most intricately designed watch. My medical education says this masterpiece was created by the trial and error of evolution. My heart says otherwise. It reveals the mind of a greater power. At every surgery, I felt humbled like an amateur painter restoring a delicate one of a kind Renaissance art masterpiece. I found it fascinating that the insides of all of us are very much alike but there are always unique quirks of anatomy, too. For this mirrors the outsides of us, too, as well as our minds and souls.

Next, I miss the people I use to worked with. I cannot put into words that would be adequate to describe them. I find it interesting there have been so many dramas, comedies, TV shows, movies and works of fiction depicting the lives and work of medical people. From M.A.S.H. through St. Elsewhere to Grey's Anatomy, doctors and nurses achieve a mythical quality, that are really not true. Some of these performances do better than others depicting what it is like working in the medical field, but none come close capture their essence.

For the extraordinary activity of medical care becomes ordinary and ordinary people do the extraordinary. For medical people are just like non-medical people. They are working to pay off the mortgage on their house. They are trying to send their children to college. They are counting the days to their next vacation. They have the same strengths and weaknesses that you have. Why these ordinary people can do the extraordinary comes from their rigorous training and years of experience. They are prepared for anything for they have seen it all before. I am guessing it is no different than other professions where ordinary people can the extraordinary where they be members of the military, the police or firefighters.

What impressed me most about my ex-coworkers were the small things. It was the ability of a group of nurses, doctors and staff to go from sitting there one minute chilling out discussing the latest gossip to coming together with a moment's notice as a cohesive team to perform a life-saving emergency cesarean section. It was the beyond tired look on the faces on night shift nurses working at 3 am knowing that after their shift they will be going home and have another full day of work raising their children. It was the encouraging and knowing look of the unspoken word from a colleague given to you before you must do a difficult surgery or delivery. It was "other world" of midnights on New Year's Eve, birthdays, Super Bowl parties and Christmases spend with your "work family."

On the other hand, there are other aspects of work that I am glad are behind me, now that I am retired. For example, that awful feeling of complete physical and mental exhaustion after a twenty-four-hour shift on call. It is combination of over-caffeination mixed with a stubby feel to your beard. It is emotional lability combined with vague mental confusion. It is photophobia to the sun when driving home afterward. It is odd food cravings at odd hours. It is the inability to stand the body odors you are emitted to yourself. It is the distant realization that you are going to have to do it all over again in just a few days.

I do not miss the pace of work. Seeing six patient an hour is everyday being Christmas Eve at Target. The difference is the customer dies if you do not do your job correctly. I will not miss the multitasking. The attempt to talk to one patient on the phone in between seeing another patient in the office at the same time worrying how your patient in the intensive care unit is doing. I do not miss the skipped meals, the binging on junk food and the interruptions of rude pharmaceutical sale people at the worst possible moment.

I will not miss the endless meetings and bureaucracy of modern medicine. You see, everything in medicine, today, is decided by a committee. Or I should say everything is discussed and *not* decided by a committee. When I was in college, one summer, I worked as an engineering aid for the federal government. I was part of a group that was responsible for buying dental supplies for the military. You cannot imagine the long and complicated process of buying some toothbrushes, toothpaste and floss. That summer turned out to be a valuable preparatory learning experience for my future medical years.

Elsewhere in this book, I have touched on how much time clinicians spend on non-clinical tasks. Complying with the demands of electronic medical records. The hoops and complexities generated by medical insurance billing. The distractions of medical-legal issues. Another big chunk of a clinician's non-clinical worktime is spent in meetings and serving on committees. Physicians spend a lot time in meetings involving both the practice they worked for and the hospital where they have privileges to practice. And at the level of the hospital, there are both committees and meetings for the entire hospital staff and at the specialty departmental level. Some committees are permanent while many others are created for a particular need.

Let me give you one example of how complex and tedious medical meetings can get. When I first entered obstetric practice in the mid-1980s, a new technique for helping a mother go into labor was discovered. This was a much-needed technology. Often the clinical situation dictates that the baby or the mother would be healthier with the baby being on the outside rather than still in the mother. The new technique, called prostaglandin cervical ripening, is a standard obstetric practice today. But it was just being accepted back then. However, the technology had been shown in multiple medical studies to be a safe and effective way to jumpstart labor. Also, multiple obstetric units in the United States and in the rest of the world were using prostaglandin ripening with much success. After doing extensive reading and research about the process, I was convinced it would be a wonderful service we could offer the mothers at our hospital. At that time, I did not understand how hospitals work. For I thought it would be a simple task to have this technique made available for our patients.

Little did I know that I would have to meet multiple times each with the chairman of the department of obstetrics, the head nurse of the delivery room and the chief pharmacist of the hospital. This was just the beginning of my journey. Reports, protocols and procedures had to be written, revised and rewritten. Multiple hospital committees had to sign off on the technique including the delivery room steering committee, the delivery room nursing policy and procedure committee and the hospital pharmacy committee. There were delays waiting for the committees to make their determinations. Then, each committee made suggestions and asked for changes so the proposal bounced around and around for over a year and half before finally being approved.

The medical meeting monster (MMM) continued to grow during my career. Let us fast forward to an example from the end of my professional working days. The hospital that employed our group of obstetricians and gynecologists felt competitive pressure from a shiny, new hospital built nearby by a competing hospital network. Like fast food restaurants and new car dealerships, hospitals will build very close to their competitors to maintain or grow their market share. For like them, hospitals survive on having a high customer (patient) volume. As we have noted earlier, this is difficult today as there is excess hospital capacity in the United States. Our hospital network responded to this perceived threat by building a new and shiny outpatient center near the new competing hospital. As part of this master defensive plan, our hospital asked our practice to be the obstetric and gynecologic staff for this new center. Although employed by the hospital, we had some independence in deciding if we wanted to be part of this new venture. Because our pay as physicians was linked to how successful we were, we wanted some financial reassurances about the risks we were taking being part of this plan.

But as we have seen time and time again, nothing is simple or quick in medicine. This topic became the center of attention at our practice meeting each week when we met as a group of physicians. It pushed aside all other concerns, including the discussion of critical patients. Scores of meetings were held between representatives of our practice and the hospital. The negotiations dragged on for over a year and a half. What became a rather simple matter of whether or not to staff a new clinic, evolved into a complete re-negotiating of our employment contracts with the hospital. The new contracts were complex and cumbersome. One needed a degree in accounting and mathematics to understand them. As a result, nerves were frayed. Harsh feelings expressed. Professional relationships hurt. Critical time was stolen from our primary duty of physicians of taking care of patients. Ironically, in the end, soon after the contracts were signed, and we began staffing the new clinic, the purpose for the new outpatient health center became obsolete. For our hospital network and the competing hospital network agreed to a merger.

The medical meeting monster is just one symptom of how highly bureaucratic American medicine is today. For example, at the time of my retirement, our practice had more non-medical workers (billers, coders, receptionists, managers) than medical ones (physicians, midlevel providers, nurses and medical assistants). On a national scale, administrative costs consume one quarter of the budgets at American hospitals. This is the highest percentage of any country in the world. Since 1970, the number of physicians in this country has doubled while the number of medical administrators has increased over thirtyfold (Woolhandler, S, Himmelstein, DU. The National Health Program Slide-Show Guide. *Center for National Health Program Studies*, Cambridge, MA, 2014.). The number of people covered by medical insurance declined by one percent between the years 2000 and 2005, but the number of people employed by medical insurance companies grew by one-third. (Krugman, P. The world of U. S. health care economics is downright scary. *Seattle Post-Intelligencer*, September 26, 2006: B1.)

All large organizations are complex systems. They must deal with the perils of their own unique bureaucracy. Whether it be a local government, a cable and internet provider or a regional bank, each has its own problems of complexities both for the organization, itself, its workers and its consumers. The general characteristics of these bureaucracies were first described by Max Weber, one of the founders of modern sociology at the turn of the twentieth century. He famously stated that bureaucracies have six defining features. They have a hierarchical structure. There are layers and layers of managers, often seen on complex organizational charts. It can seem like everyone working at one is a "middle manager." Second, there are lots and lots of rules that define the organization's policies and procedures. Third, there is a rigid division of labor. Jobs are tightly defined and not much flexibility in their descriptions. Fourth, workers advance their position within the bureaucracy based upon how well they do their job. Fifth, such organizations work towards efficacy of their operations. Finally, bureaucracies create impersonal environments. As you can see from these definitions, bureaucracies are not necessarily bad, and there certainly are not avoidable workplace structures. But one of the fundamental goals, as we create our new SPUN Healthcare system, is both to eliminate the weaknesses of our present system and prevent from creating new ones with our future one.

Why does are our present healthcare system have such bureaucratic problems and are the possible solutions? The biggest contributor to today's system complexities is our multiple payer system. There are several different governmental payers and dozens of private insurers. Each has several different plans that are continually shifting over time. That means there are hundreds of different rule sets for the healthcare system. That, in turn, creates the need for a complex organization to create, write, enforce, interpret and understand the rules. Such a bureaucracy is needed both on the insurer side and the provider side. One side is making and enforcing the rules. The other side is interpreting and complying to them.

The solution to this complexity is simple. Having one payer with one set of rules for everyone in the country, not only would provide universal, less expensive healthcare, it will be a much more efficient system. Do you want proof? Countries, such as Canada, that have a single payer system, but private hospitals and other medical providers have much lower administrative overhead that the United States.

Second, a medical provider, whether they be a rural dentist working for himself or the Mayo Clinic, is beholden to a complex set of regulations at the local, state and federal level. These rules are conflicting, overlapping or redundant. Plus, they must be reconciled with the medical insurance rules. As described earlier, having the SPUN National Health System in charge of all aspects of healthcare regulation in the country would create a single regulatory structure. This is another example of having just one set of rules for everyone to follow that would lead to simplicity.

Third, we do not have a national system of medical records. In fact, several different record systems inhabit the same hospital or medical organization. Therefore, the biggest wonder of efficiency in the last thirty years, the near instant transfer of information anywhere in the world, has bypassed American medicine. Even those online medical records that do exist are fundamentally flawed. They exist more to serve to the purposes of third-party insurance payers and the medico-legal system than the informational needs of healthcare providers and patients.

Besides being inefficient, such a scattered system of healthcare records leads to higher medical costs, redundant medical testing, lost opportunities for early diagnosis and treatment of disease, a lost research opportunity to mine all the country's healthcare data to improve future healthcare and contributes mightily to provider burnout. A universal set of healthcare records that are designed for the needs of providers and patients will be an instant red tape slasher of the American healthcare bureaucracy.

Fourth, we need clinicians to focus on clinical work. When a family physician is spending time on insurance billing, when a hospital nurse is doing staffing and scheduling, when an emergency room physician is trying to track down a blood test performed on a patient elsewhere a week ago or when an orthopedic surgeon is scheduling surgery, that means there is that much less time for patient care. We need more healthcare workers' time in the trenches doing the basic medical work of diagnosing and treating. We already have seen as the proposed SPUN Healthcare Plan can simplify the process of billing and retrieving medical information. We have proposed a new clerical assistant role to aid medical providers in performing non-clinical tasks. Healthcare organizations need to do their part, too. They need to look at all the non-clinical tasks their clinicians perform and move as many as possible to non-clinicians.

Fifth, medical care roles are too rigid. As we have seen, this is an unfortunate consequence of a bureaucracy. No human endeavor has as many different types of workers and professions as medicine. A typical hospital has hundreds of different nurse specialties, laboratory workers, equipment technologists, therapists, social workers, insurance specialists and physician specialties. Each have defined roles of what they can but also what they cannot do. This can foster a trades mentality. Everyone is afraid to do anything that might not be in their job description. I saw examples of this every day when I was practicing medicine. A physician will not push a button of a patient's intravenous pump and turn off the annoying beeping indicating an infusion is complete. Resident physicians receive so much training in their specialty, but they never learn the simple task how to draw blood on a patient. Nurses are forbidden to give patients critical test results. Specialists, making rounds in the hospital, concentrate so much on their own field, they do not know the primary reason the patient was admitted to the hospital in the first place.

Hospitals, physician practices and other healthcare systems preach teamwork but put up roadblocks from allowing it to happen. When I was first in practice, there was a surgeon nicknamed "Hoppy." Hoppy was not afraid to do any task for his patient. You would see him wheeling his patient on a stretcher back to the operating room when an orderly was not available. He would carry critical pathology specimens down to the laboratory from the operating room to be read. Instead of drinking coffee in the physician's lounge between surgical cases, he would help clean the operating room, even mopping the floor. Today, Hoppy would have his wings clipped. The hospital would cite a thousand insurance and legal reasons that would prevent him from helping on these non-surgical tasks.

No, I am not saying your dentist should prescribe your eye glass prescription or your pharmacist be your psychotherapist. However, our future SPUN licensure system will allow much more flexibility in what each medical profession can do. In addition, healthcare organizations from the smallest rural solo practice to the largest hospital system should run with an empowerment concept instilled into its workers. Empowerment is a wonderful thing. Not only would it make healthcare less bureaucratic, more personal and less costly, it would release the full potential of its workers.

Sixth, we must get rid of the "gray-haired wiseman (or wise woman)" syndrome in healthcare. Medical practice is extremely hierarchal. Take a hospital's physician staff, for example. At the bottom rung are the medical students. Above them are residents in training with each year's residents reporting to one a year ahead of them. Next come fellows in subspecialty training. Finally, at the top of the organizational pyramid, there is the attending physician. Even among attendings, critical decisions usually are deferred to the oldest and supposedly wisest (and usually the grayest) member of that group. Experience trumps novelty. The one with the most degrees beats out the one with the best thinking. Thinking gets conservative, if not ossified. On hospital rounds, it is entertaining to see this group march through the building, virtually in single file with the attending physician being the drum major and the medical student trying not to be left too far behind. Information and communications flow like it does in the military. It moves through each link of the chain of command like a game of whisper down the line.

To solve the problem of the gray-haired wiseman, we need a cultural change in medicine. Our SPUN National Healthcare Plan will not be able to fix this problem its own. Decision-making in medicine must be more collaborative rather than so authoritative. The best idea does not necessarily come from the top of the chain of command or from the oldest member of a team or necessary from a physician. The automaker, Toyota, became a top car seller with a deserved reputation for quality because it had a different culture than other manufacturers. It famously allowed the lowest assembly line workers to put the switch and stop the entire production line if they saw a problem. Medicine will benefit from that kind of thinking.

Seventh, medical systems must revise their complex organizational structure. That means change means more than getting rid of an excessive of non-medical middle managers. (Although that would be a helpful first step.) Medical structural organization is too much by profession and not enough by functioning units. For example, in a typical American hospital, there is a physician staff and a nursing staff. The physician staff is organized by specialty such as surgery and obstetrics/gynecology. The nursing staff is organized by departments, including the operating room and the delivery room. That does not make sense. For surgeons are working very closely with the nursing staff in the operating room and the obstetrician/gynecologists work with closely with the nursing staff in the delivery room. Yet they are in two separate organizational structures. Instead of having two parallel ones with much overlap and possibly competing goals, they should be combined into one.

Let us start with the example of the delivery room. The obstetric nurses and the obstetricians will be on one team. Anesthesiologists and neonatologists would also be part of this new integrated department. There will be one set of rules for all. Problems that cropped up will be addressed by this one department rather than bounce back and forth between nursing and physician. In addition to being more efficient in solving problems, it will foster better communications among the healthcare workers who are working closely together. Since everyone in a certain area of a hospital is working for the same group, it would promote teamwork among the group of different professionals.

Similarly, operating room nurses, scrub technicians, general surgeons, the various specialty surgeons, anesthesiologists and nurse anesthetics will be organized in a single operating room department. Note that different workers could be on more than one team. For example, anesthesiologists would be both in the operating room department and the delivery room department.

This rethinking of organizing medical workers by functional groups rather than by professions will extend to the office or outpatient setting. Back when I was in practice, on days that I was working the office, my family could tell which medical assistant that I had worked with that day by the mood I was in when I walked in the door from work. For each day in the office, medical assistants, office receptionists and physicians, each from separate divisions of the practice, were randomly assigned to work together for that day. Because this group had to work so closely together for that day, but the composition of the group was always changing, the group never had a chance to coalesce as team. Therefore, it was just a matter of chance if team functioned well that day (I came home from work happy.) or functioned poorly (My children hid in their bedroom when I walked in the house.). The solution was obvious, set office work groups. Organize a big practice by creating a bunch of little ones. Each consists of small teams that work together even though their jobs are different. This will create a team rather than just a bunch of people working together. For a team is more than the sum of its parts. A team will more efficient and work for a common goal. A team will allow for experimentation and innovation of how things were done. A team will create new efficiencies in the way things are done. A team will give a large medical practice, a small practice feel. For what we want in medicine is the nice touches of the corner drug store with the conveniences and prices of CVS. We want the personal feel of the mom and pop hardware store with the selection of The Home Depot. Most American healthcare takes place in large medical practices, hospitals and clinics. They are way too impersonal. A team approach to these health settings will capture some of that Norman Rockwell we all crave.

Eighth, medical systems must rethink how and when they use meetings and committees. This gets us back to the lead-in at the start of this chapter. I recognize that the medical meeting monster is everywhere in modern bureaucracies, not just in medicine. Still, hospitals have too many standing committees. And these committees meet too often even if there is not any significant purpose for that meeting. For once a committee is formed in medicine, it has a life of its own. It would be better if committees were formed and met to serve one specific function, solve that problem and then dissolve. Think back to my example with the prostaglandin gel. Instead of the issue bouncing back and forth among several different committees, each with partial interest and decision power, a unique committee should have been formed to decide if and how this medication was going to be used. After two or three meetings, the issue would have been resolved and that committee ended.

Many medical meetings are designed just to give information to employees. Often an hour's worth of fifty workers' time is used in such a meeting that could have been replaced with a simple email. Often medical meetings are more like a group therapy session or happy hour after work on Friday afternoons. There is a lot of idle talk, mindless whining and complaining and tales of old medical war stories. Typically, the traditional meeting rules are not followed. Discussion is scattered. There is no set time limit. They do not start on time. Members arrive late, come and go as they please during the meeting and are not engage with the meeting as it is occurring. Sometimes, there is not even a formal agenda.

Medical meetings are too big. They have too many participants. Jeffrey Bezos, the founder and head of Amazon, said a meeting should not have more members than can be fed with two pizzas. Instead, today's medical meetings and committees have dozens and dozens of members. In a showy attempt to be democratic, everyone and anyone is invited to participate. As a result, these meetings use up a lot of valuable time of its members. Physicians, in particular, are control freaks. As much as they hate non-medical tasks, especially meetings, they despise even more not being included as part of the decision-making process. For it can be a badge of honor to serve on certain medical committees. Meetings with such large number of members are unwieldy. With a large group, it can be hard to form a consensus. Discussion is dominated by just a few people. The smaller the group, the faster a decision can be made.

Also, there needs to be a lead person from the committee to take sole ownership of the problem at hand. That person will be responsible for steering the committee to reach a final and definite decision. For group ownership of a problem usually means no ownership. Along this line, there should be a defined time limit for making the decision. When matters are left open-ended, there often is no end. Even if you do not work not in medicine, you probably recognize these committee and meeting problems occur in your field, too. Just because it is a universal problem, does not mean it cannot be solved. For American medicine can go a long way to slay the bureaucratic monster it created by controlling the number, size, scope, efficiency and organization of its meetings and committees.

Ninth, American medicine needs to standardize and simplify its many complex tasks using checklists. Have you ever planned a wedding, surprise party or other large gathering of people? It can be overwhelming to coordinate the music, food, venue and guest lists. One misstep, say forgetting to order the ice, and the event can be a flop. To prevent such missteps, you surely used a checklist of what had to be done and in what order. The practice of medicine is very similar. For much of what happens in healthcare can be likened to planning for a party. For you must gather a group of people at the same place and same time with the necessary supplies and equipment for a particular goal. Even as seemingly simple a task as sending someone home from the hospital involves the scheduling of outpatient follow-up appointments, getting necessary prescription medication and other medical supplies for the patient, providing transportation home, billing concerns and coordination of future home care. Think of the medical team that must be coordinated and the equipment and supplies needed for the ordinary hospital task of a patient having surgery to have her gallbladder removed. Having so many complex and multistep tasks in medicine opens up the system for missteps. At the very least, these missteps cause a waste of time and money. All too often, they lead to serious but preventable patient complications.

American medicine has taken some cues from the aviation and other non-medical industries to simplify the organization of these complex tasks by the using checklists. Before an airplane can take off, it must be thoroughly checked out by the flight crew. Standardized checklists have been developed to make sure these checks are completed. Huge manuals of checklists exist for the spaceflights and in the nuclear power industry, covering routine situations and possible emergencies. The "timeout" is a recent example in medicine of using this checklist philosophy. Before a surgery or other procedure can begin, a checklist is reviewed to make sure all the needed personnel and equipment are at the ready. Also, any tasks that were needed to be completed for the procedure are checked off for completeness. The timeout has a valuable psychologic benefit, too. It gives the team a chance to focus on the upcoming task and make sure everyone is on the same page as to what will happen. Sometimes members of the team do not even know one another, and this time allows for simple introductions. It can create a sense of a team in the operating room or the clinic. The start of operations can be chaotic as there are many people and much equipment gathered in a small space. Many people are talking at once or running around in different directions. The time out can create a needed sense of calm at the beginning. This calmness is beneficial both for the team to focus and for the patient to be less fearful.

Let me give you another example of this checklist philosophy. At the delivery room where I used to work, they had several printed checklists posted throughout the department. These checklists were step by step instructions for what to do in case of several serious obstetric emergencies. They included information for life-threatening complications of epidural anesthesia, for neonatal resuscitation, for shoulder dystocia (when the baby's shoulders get stuck in the maternal pelvis after the baby's head has delivered) and for maternal hemorrhage after delivery. We all need "cheat-cheats" from time to time. Especially, when our emotions start to get the best of us during a critical situation. Plus, having the print-ups prominently around the department meant that they continuously being read and the information absorbed by the obstetric team. That made all of us better prepared for the next crisis. The checklists also acted as a security blanket. Just knowing that they were there gave you confidence ahead of time if trouble should brew.

Medicine needs more of these emergency checklists available. Common ones should be printed and displayed on the walls of our hospitals, offices and clinics, like they were in my old hospital's delivery room. Less common ones will be part of the SPUN EMR system, so a team member can refer to it on a computer screen in a moment's notice should the situation occur. For often what is most lifesaving devise in a critical situation is not a million-dollar piece of equipment but a simple piece of paper.

There will be checklists for non-emergency situations, too. And such checklists will have ownership for their completion. As mentioned above, it can be so hard for a patient to get discharged out of a hospital or emergency room. This leads to needless delays. Plus, it ties up a hospital bed causing delays in treating other patients. All this adds costs for our healthcare system. A simple checklist for checkout, managed ("owned") by the patient's nurse or a specialized discharge planner will expedite the process. As a second example, diabetic patients need a lot of continuing monitoring for possible complications of the disease. Their hemoglobin A1c, a blood test that monitors how well their blood sugars are being controlled needs to be performed periodically. Their heart, eyes, kidney function and even their feet should be checked, on a regular basis. To make sure these screening tasks are being completed, a popup checklist will appear on the electronic medical record of the diabetic patient when she is being seen by the physician who is primarily responsible for her care. The patient, too, will have the same popup list on her health app to encourage her to take more ownership of her own health.

Unlike what you see on television medical dramas, emergencies are not occurring every second of every day in our hospitals. Most of the time, things are going according to plan and care is routine. But when medical crises do happen, the staff must be prepared and be prepared for dozens of different possibilities. The best way to prepare everyone for all these scenarios is by drills. Think about it for a moment. The military continually drills for different war game scenarios. Fire departments drill for different types of fire emergencies. Police drill in a similar manner. School practice fire drills (and unfortunately in our modern world, lockdown drills). And what are pre-seasons and practice sessions for sports teams but a series of drills? Therefore, it is common sense that medical teams drill for both common and uncommon emergencies that can occur in their department.

These checklists and drills, by themselves, will not be enough. Medicine must simplify as much as possible, its complex processes. It has too many forms. It has too much paperwork. There are too many steps to do simple things. For with more steps, there is more complexity. With more complexity, the more likely errors can occur. Emphasis is taken away from the primary goal of patient safety. Have you ever been to an old building that gradually has been added upon over the years? If you look carefully, you can see wings and additions built on to a tiny main structure. On the inside, ceilings and floors of the various parts do not exactly meet. The rooms do not flow one to another in a functional matter. Instead, a bedroom might be next to the kitchen. Interestingly, most hospitals are built on the same addon design. Wings and additions and remodels are attached to a small, ancient structure. On the inside, there is a confusing and disordered organization to where different departments are located. For example, at the hospital where I used to work, the postpartum area was divided into two different areas, located in two different buildings, and both far from the labor and delivery suite. No, this is not a lost page from an introduction to a course in architecture. For what is true in old building hospital design, is true in hospital procedures. Tasks and protocols are continually added on to an original procedure creating a complex and confusing formula for how things are done.

Of course, you cannot do go and build new a completely new hospital building from scratch, every time it needs some more room. But you can build new procedures and protocols from scratch, when you need to make changes. Let me give you a simple example. Every time the legal department or governmental regulations demanded a new consent form, it was created and *added* to the pile that the patient (usually does not read and) signs. That is part of the reason why you have that pile. Instead, we could have *one* form with all the information that is needed for the consent. The goal should be when there is the need for one new piece of paper, it should replace (at least) two. If a new step is added to a process, it should replace two. And the best way of achieving this simplification is by recreating the wheel.

A common office procedure in a gynecologist's office is placing an IUD (intrauterine device) inside a patient's uterine for contraception. Every time one needed to be placed, I would see the medical assistant that I was working with run around the office on a bizarre scavenger hunt, looking for all the necessary equipment for the procedure. What a waste of time and efficiency with the possible room for error if a critical tool was missing. Again, the solution is simple. Create preassembled kits, with all the necessary equipment, ahead of time.

One huge area of complexity in medicine that is in desperate need of simplification is the "handoff." You guessed it. It is named after the football play, when the quarterback hands the football to a running back. Like the football play, it is a common time in medicine for peril. For fumbles happen. In medicine, the handoff is when the care of a patient is transferred from one medical caretaker to another. It typically involves either the nursing and physician care. Handoffs happen during a change of shift, to redistribute the caretaker's workload and during vacations, meals and breaks. During the handoff, the outgoing provider gives a summary report of the patient's case to an incoming provider. The problem with this situation is the same problem with the game "whisper down the line." Critical information is not passed on. Emphasis on important parts of the case is not made. The incoming provider is overwhelmed with a vast amount of information and cannot assimilate it all. The problem is compounded when there are multiple handoffs on the same patient. It is not unusual for a laboring mother to have a dozen or more different nurses take care of her during her labor and delivery.

The handoff is becoming even more of an issue, today. There are work rules now for physician interns and residents. Unlike in the bad old days, there are legal limits on how many hours in a row a physician in training can work. This means more handoffs and therefore, more possibilities for error. This is ironic because the work rules were created to improve patient care and safety by not having sleepy physicians rendering medical care. The creation of more handoff is why such an expected reduction in errors from work rules has not occurred.

Ask any medical professional and they will tell you they never know the cases of patients whom they received in handoffs as well as those they have taken care of from the beginning. One of the common scary moments for me in medical practice was when I was called from office hours to deliver a patient's baby because my covering partner was busy. Walking into a delivery at the last possible second, knowing nothing about the case, was very unsettling to say the least. One of the riskiest times in the hospital to be a patient is dinnertime. The usual staff of physicians taking care of the patient is gone for the day. They have handed off the care to the call group for the night. The call group has not gotten an adequate familiarity with the patient, yet. At the same time, there is a new nursing staff taking care of the patient as the typical time of nursing change of shift is 3 pm. And to make matters worse, there is a third covering nurse as new evening shift nurse has gone off for a dinner break. Therefore, if an emergency arises during this time, there is no one there who truly understands the total picture of what is going on.

The best solution to the handoff problem is to reduce the number of times that it happens. Just like in football, the less times the ball is transferred from one player to another, the less chance of a fumble. The same philosophy applies to medicine. I am not advocating for longer shift hours. This will not work, either. For example, take the nursing staff. Studies show the error rate in patient care goes up after eight-hour shift length. (K. Reid and D. Dawson, "Comparing Performance on Simulated Twelve Hour Shift Rotation in Young and Older Subjects," Occupational and Environmental Medicine 58, no. 1 (2001): 58–62) Rather every effort should be made to keep the same patient with the same care provider.

Second, the handoffs should be staggered as much as possible. This can be accomplished by varying the break times in a department. Also, physician and nursing handoffs should be different so there is always someone on board who has some experience with the patient.

Third, the information for the handoff should be standardized. A concise but formal dataset for the passage of the football of care will make a fumble less likely.

Fourth, it should be clear to the patient and to all other caretakers who is taking care of the patient. Some hospitals now have chalkboards in patients' room with this information. Our SPUN EMR will note on the patient's record who is in charge at every level of care and it should be updated every time a handoff occurs.

Finally, there should be more of a team aspect to medical care. For example, having two nurses take care of ten patients might be better than one nurse taking care of five. If one nurse gets extra busy with one patient or takes a meal break, there still is another nurse available who knows the patient's case.

The handoff problem *within* a medical facility is a serious enough problem. A more complicated one is the handoff problem *between* facilities or practices. That is, what happens when your care is divided up among different hospitals, the hospital and the outpatient setting and among different physicians of different specialties. This is such a critical problem that it requires a whole chapter to discuss, the subject of the next one.

10. WHO WILL BE IN CHARGE?

Online shopping is such a convenience. Sometimes we forget that this technology has been around for only a couple of decades. Search, point, click from anywhere just with your phone and what you want is on your front doorstep in a couple of days. Books, computers, electronics, toys, clothes, food and even cars appear like magic. Yes, Virginia, you were right. Santa Claus is real. Today, Amazon reigns supreme for this online shopping experience. Here you can find almost anything. And if you have their special Prime Membership, it is delivered in two days or less. But one thing that you may not know about Amazon is that over half of the items sold from the website do not come from the company, itself (Statista website, data from the second quarter 2018). Instead, they come from third-party vendors who use the Amazon website to sell their wares. Over two million different sellers sell two billion items here each year. It is a great system for everyone. Amazon gets a cut of every item sold. The seller gets the exposure of Amazon. For it is an opportunity for a small retailer to sell their items anywhere in the world. All of us buying stuff get a greater variety of items, at one convenient online location. The interesting thing about this online shopping experience is that it feels like you are buying from just one company. You could be purchasing ten items from the site, five from Amazon, itself, and five more from four different vendors. But you just have to checkout and pay one bill. If you have a problem with any of the items, whether sold by Amazon or by one of its outside vendors, there is just one place you must go to have it sorted out. Why am I discussing Amazon? Our healthcare system should emulate the company.

To completely mix my metaphors, I want our SPUN Healthcare Insurance to encourage a general home builder system for how we deliver medical care in the United States. For when you want to put an addition on your house, you hire just one contractor. That person hires or "subs out" in the trade lingo, the electrical work, plumbing, drywalling and painting to the "specialists." They do most of the actual work of the building your addition. But the work is supervised and overseen by the general contractor. He is the one person that you pay and the one you go to with any complaints about the quality of the work being performed. Just as the in case of Amazon, the subcontractors work independently of each other and of the general contractor.

Here is yet another critical element missing in medicine. An adult in charge. Let me give you a hypothetical example but it will be one that I am sure will be familiar to you. Let us say you have an annoying cough. You have had it now for several months. You have tried waiting it out and have tried some over the counter therapies without any relief. You and your spouse are losing sleep, every night, because of it. You both are scared you have something serious. But mostly, you just want it to go away. Finally, desperate for some help, you make an appointment to see your family physician. Of course, you cannot see *your* doctor. She is too busy, so you get an appointment with her associate who, of course, you have never met. It is an awkward visit for both of you. It is frustrating having your care provided by someone who knows nothing about it. Although this associate physician seems nice enough, it is hard to build the needed rapport in just a few minutes. It also feels like reinventing the wheel for the fill-in doctor. He knows nothing about your medical history. Feeling a constant time pressure as he is always being behind schedule, he must review as much of the gigabytes of medical data about you on his electronic medical record as he can in as short amount of time as possible. Plus, he is multitasking while seeing you. He is answering phone calls from other patients, getting sidelined by pharmaceutical salespeople in the hallway and worrying about the patient he saw one hour ago that he had to send to the emergency room in an ambulance. In the examination room, the pinch-hit doctor takes a brief history from you and listens to your chest as you breathe. He concludes it is just a "viral thing" and gives you a prescription for a cough medication. After waiting an hour in a busy chain store pharmacy, catching up on People magazine, you finally get your medication and go home. You start taking the medication, hoping to feel better.

One week goes by. Then two. Although you are not getting worse, you are not getting any better either. You still have the nagging cough which is keeping you up all night. So, you call your family doctor's office again looking for advice. They can't help you. Instead, the staff insists that you come back into the office for another consultation. You first are reluctant as you do not want to miss another day at work. But you finally agree to be seen. At least, your appointment is with your regular physician, which required a bit of begging and a lot of negotiating. Your appointment with her is much more comfortable than was the one with her associate. She asks about your family and job and even remembers your children's names. She, too, is more comfortable with you. You can surmise this because she does not keep looking at her laptop computer with a lost-look stare on her face. Her assessment of your cough is that you have a minor case of pneumonia. She gives you a prescription for an antibiotic, wants you to get a chest x-ray and have some blood work performed. Disney Land time. You finish the People magazine you started a month ago at the pharmacy. You miss yet another half of day of work, waiting for the ten seconds to get your chest x-ray taken and having bloodwork drawn.

You take the new medication, but you still do not improve. It also is unnerving that you have not heard the results from your tests. You start to worry that you have some deadly disease. In a panic, you call your family doctor's office. After navigating the office's phone tree, waiting on hold several times and dealing with rude receptionists, you talk with the triage nurse. You find out from her that your chest x-ray and blood work are normal. But she is not willing to give you and more advice about what to do about your cough, other than make another appointment with the office. Frustrated, angry and demanding, you insist on speaking with your doctor. One day goes by. And another and you have not heard from the office. Finally, you see the office's phone appear on your phone as it rings. But you let out a heavy sigh when you answer the phone and hear the voice on the other end. It is the *first* doctor that you saw for the cough. The pinch-hit one. Although he is professional, he is not helpful, because he is not your doctor. He offers to leave a message for your physician to get back to you. Another day passes, and the cough is not any better. The Murphy's Law of Medicine takes hold. It states that the most critical phone call from your doctor will come at the worst possible time. It does, as you are in the middle of a work meeting with your boss. This is followed by a game of phone tag between you and your doctor over the next two days.

After the expected exchange of pleasantries, you discuss your persistent cough with her. She seems both surprised and stumped. She suggests that you get a CT scan and see a lung specialist, a pulmonologist. CT scan? Lung specialist? Now you are *really* scared and even go as far as checking the terms of your life insurance policy. You journey through Disney Land will get longer. For not only will you be seeing the pulmonologist about your persistent cough, but also will be seeing an allergist, an eye nose and throat specialist and a gastrointestinal specialist. At each specialist's office, you must deal with phone trees, unhelpful receptionists, long waits for appointments, redundant paperwork, repeat physical examinations and more testing. You meet all types of physicians. Some are nice. Others, you can tell, make you feel like you are wasting their time. None are all that helpful. All they say is that it is the organ of yours that they examine, and test is normal. But you want to know what is *wrong*. Each ends their relationship with you by either bouncing you back to family doctor or suggesting yet another specialist for you to see. Throughout the many evaluations, you are confused as to who to call for results or advice. Such bouncing around Disney Land from ride to ride is frustrating when you are healthy. But remember, you are not feeling that great. You have this nagging cough. You are not sleeping well at night. You are missing so work and are feeling the pressure from your boss and from your family. Finally, like the proverbial lost object that is not found until you look in the final spot, the last physician you see, the gastrointestinal specialist, figures out the cause of your cough. You have severe gastro-intestinal reflux that is the trigger for it. He puts you on an acid blocking medication and your cough goes away in a couple of days.

I am sure this story sounds familiar. That you, a family member or friend has had a similar tale or tales. In fact, it is the most common story I hear when I am out socially when I meet someone new and they find out I am a physician. They related to me a long tale of frustration. That no one had ownership of their health problem. The medical wanderings they went through to finally get an answer. Whether it be for a cough, headache, abdominal pain, insomnia, depression or heart palpitations, the tale of woe is similar. The story is worse when that someone has a chronic or serious disease, like a cancer or an auto-immune disorder. For example, a breast cancer patient sees a minimum of five physicians for her disease. That list includes a surgeon, a medical oncologist, radiation oncologist, gynecologist and a family physician. Can you see the problem? Who does she call first if she has a question or concern? Plus, when she receives conflicting advice, who does she believe?

What our healthcare system needs is a point person for each of your healthcare problems. Someone in charge. A general contractor who can coordinate the care of the subcontractors. A single practitioner in complete control of the care for that problem. One physician in one practice. Let us go back to your chronic cough problem and rerun the tape as it should have played. When you first contacted your family physician with the chronic cough, every effort should have been made by that office for you to see her. It is just common sense that you see the one physician who knows you best. Then, when your family physician sees you, she lists a new problem in your medical record. This automatically is added to your problem list. The term, problem list, is exactly what it sounds like, a list of all your health concerns. That includes both ongoing ones, like hypertension and time-limited ones, like a case of influenza. Problem lists, in medicine, like problems in life in general are fluid. Some come and go, and others never go away. The problem with problem lists (pun intended), today, is that no one practitioner has ownership of the each of the problems on the list.

That was what happened in the case of your cough. The responsibility for the management of it bounced around different practitioners and other members of the staff of both your family physician's office and the various specialists. What should have happened is that your personal family physician had total ownership of your problem, until the very end when it was discovered to be reflux disease. Then, the problem baton would have been passed off to the gastrointestinal specialist. It will be an easy matter to make sure that a practitioner has ownership of all your medical problems. When a new problem is created in your medical record, that clinician has ownership of it. The mere act of entering a new problem in the electronic medical record system will give ownership of it to that practitioner. That physician or midlevel provider oversees its management. There is clearly defined responsibility.

You may argue that practitioners might not want to take on such health problem ownership. After all, who wants ownership of more troubles? That medical problems could become hot potatoes, rapidly passed from one healthcare provider to another. That is the beauty of the proposed SPUN Healthcare Plan payment system. Since *all* time a practitioner spends taking care of a patient is billable time, practitioners will be happy to be in charge since it means more money in their pockets. In the future, overseeing a patient's problem will be an advantage to the physician, not a disadvantage as it is today.

What will it mean to be in charge of a patient's problem? That practitioner will be the point person. She will be the one medical provider that patient goes to with all his questions, concerns and follow up care. That provider will be in charge of the medical management, review all test results and coordinate all care outside of her practice.

For hospitalized patients, this means a stronger role for the admitting physician. Today, the attending physician often is just one of several providers taking care of one part of you when you are in the hospital. Often, no one seems to take command of your case. Instead, the admitting physician will coordinate the care of all the specialists and consultants seeing you. She will have the holistic view of you and medical care. That will take a change of thinking for most physicians. For we are usually more lone wolfs than team players. In our medical training, we need more lessons on working as both part of a team and being a leader of a team.

We cannot keep going into hospitals, take care of one organ of our patients and leave. Instead, we need playground skills of communication, building consensus and harmony and taking turns being the captain of the team.

Let us take this concept one step further. Each of us needs someone in charge of all our health concerns. Someone who can coordinate the medical care of all the health problems on our medical record list. Someone who realizes that your new onset headaches might be the result of problems at work or the stress of dealing with your mother's worsening dementia. Someone who can see all the connections and conflicts in your life. That provider should be your primary care provider. Whether it be a family care physician, internist, gynecologist, pediatrician or midlevel provider, that role needs more emphasis on the total ownership of a patient's care. Today, unfortunately, too many primary care providers are like busy receptionists in the lobby of large office buildings. They are great at directing you where to go when you need specialized care, but their ownership of your healthcare ends when they pass you on to them.

Why did that happen? How did primary care physicians lose ownership of the complete package of healthcare that is you? There are lots of reasons. The science of medicine has become more complicated. It is ever changing. Therefore, it is impossible for one physician to know it all or keep up with it all. As a result, today is the age of specialists and subspecialists. They are practitioners who know more and more about very specialized fields and tiny wedges of medical knowledge. Not only are there more neurologists but more neurologists who specialize in headaches and headache specialists who concentrate on cluster headaches and so on and so on. Second, the huge student loan debt that newly minted physicians carry encourages them to go into the higher paying specialties and subspecialties and shun primary care medicine. Third, there is an unfortunate attitudinal problem in medicine. Too many specialists look down their noses at primary care physicians. They mock that primaries do not know as much about *their* specialty as they do. Of course, that is absurd. A general contractor need only know the basics of roofing to direct and understand a roofer. The same is true for the relationship between a primary care physician and a specialist. Fourth, as we have seen, there is a communication problem among all physicians. They are reluctant to talk to one another. Because specialists do not communicate directly with primary care physicians often enough, they do not understand their unique knowledge base and skills.

Finally, the introduction of hospitalists into today's practice of medicine has fragmented our healthcare delivery system even more. For it creates its own ownership problems. In the not too distant past in the history of American healthcare, your primary care physician was the attending doctor in charge of your case when you were admitted to the hospital. At the very least, he was a consultant on the case. Today, that role has been taken over by hospitalists. They are primary care doctors, who only practice in the hospital and manage your care just while you are hospitalized. They are so entrenched in the practice of American medicine, today, other specialties are considering moving to the hospitalist model. For example, my old specialty, obstetrics, unfortunately is on its way to such a system. This is how it would work. When you are pregnant, your prenatal care will be given by one set of obstetricians. Then your labor and delivery care will be administered by another group. I am not questioning that hospitalists do not give excellent care. But there is a very real danger with such a model. Our healthcare needs are getting further fragmented, especially in the role of who oversees all of you.

How can primary care physicians regain their vital general contractor role? First, primary care residencies, the on the job training period, need to be longer. Today, family medicine, internal medicine and general pediatric residencies are the shortest of all the specialties. There is just three years of training after medical school. One or two additional years would prepare future primary care doctors for their complex role in coordinating healthcare. Second, primary care physician's salaries should be in line with that of the specialists. Future physicians chose their specialties for the same reason Willy Sutton robbed banks. Because that is where the money is, and today, it is in the specialties. To attract more of the best and brightest, society should pay primary care doctors at a significantly higher rate than it does today. SPUN's system of lower student debt also will help future physicians from picking the specialty fields with higher pay but less need.

Third, all physicians should talk to each other more often. Primary care physicians need to talk more to the specialists that are taking care of their patients. A doctor sending a patient with a slip a paper or a pile of lab reports to another doctor is not really communication. A specialist sending a letter back to the primary physician, two weeks after the consultation is not truly communication. We must stop making the patient the messenger traveling back and forth between primary care doctor and specialist, relaying critical medical information. A simple phone call would help the specialist understand both the patient she is about to see and the primary doctor's concerns about her. The phone call would help the primary care provider have ownership of the patient and the case and demonstrate to the specialist her competency and responsibility.

A universal set of medical records, as proposed for the SPUN system, also will be a huge step forward. Since all the information that the specialist sees is in the same chart system as what the primary sees, communication, coordination and ownership of care will be enhanced. Finally, American medicine should seriously rethink the role and the necessity of the hospitalist physician. Is the advantage of having such specialized physicians who just do the work of taking take of patients in the hospital worth the risk of the further fragmentation of patient care that exists today?

The problem of the ownership of patients' health concerns goes beyond the medical profession. Americans, unfortunately, have gotten use to someone doing all their thinking and legwork for them. We think that by paying someone to advise us, we do not have to do any of the work, ourselves. We will pay an accountant to do our income taxes, though our tax situation is simple, and our tax return is just one page. Thus, we do not understand our personal finances. We will pay a stock broker high brokerage fees to manage our retirement savings, although all we need to a low fee index mutual fund. Thus, we do not understand our investments. We will pay a lawyer to fight our traffic ticket, when we could have could fought it ourselves. The same holds true for our health needs and that of our families. We think since we pay for health services (and pay a lot), we do not feel the need to be involved in our own medical care.

When I practiced medicine, I saw pathetic examples of lack of healthcare ownership, every day. Patients did not know the names of the medications they took on a regular basis or even why they took them. Patients had surgeries that did not know the reason why they were performed. Patients knew little about their family history. Diabetic patients knew next to nothing about their disease, its control or complications. Hypertensive patients did not know what their blood pressure readings typically ran. Patients lacked basic information about what constitutes a healthy diet or the importance of being physically active. This dangerous naivety that I witnessed crossed all boundaries. It was independent of the race, intelligence, education or profession of the patient.

Why is it important? When patients are involved in their own healthcare, they are more compliant with its needs and treatment and as a result, they are much healthier. Our future healthcare plan must encourage us to take ownership of our own bodies and minds. Having access to all our medical records in one spot is an important first step. The SPUN universal medical record app for patients will provide all this information. Instead of multiple patient online portals with long forgotten user names and passwords, piles of medication information sheets from the pharmacy mixed in with discount coupons and a ragged accordion file filled with lab reports and medical insurance receipts, all the medical information that a patient will ever need will be here. The interface will provide a summary of the patient's medical problems, both ongoing and acute. Lists of medications, allergies, surgeries and past history will be easily accessible. There will be no need to track down the results of medical tests either from the past week or the past decade. The app will make them accessible from any computer or smartphone.

One of the problems of our information age is determining which information is legitimate and what is "fake news." From Google's point of view, the random and mad musings of a crackpot appear to have the same validity as a research report from the New York Times. What is true for politics and world news, is true for medical information, too. When a patient "googles" their symptoms or disease, they get hundreds of links which may lead to excellent facts and advice or wrong and dangerous information. Today's patients have little guide as to what is correct or what is not. The SPUN portal will make it easier for the patient to get legitimate information about their health as it will link directly to sites written or reviewed by its own medical experts.

The SPUN patient portal also will make it easier for patients to communicate directly with those in charge of their health. Whether it is a specialist for a specific disease or a primary care physician for an overall concern, the system will have multiple means of contact, including messaging, texting, emailing and phoning. This will enhance that critical partnership of patient and physician.

Our SPUN EMR app also can actively promote patient's health and encourage positive behaviors. Earlier in this book, we talked about how it can remind patients to take their medications and schedule routine health screenings. It can send the patients reminders to do simple but important health-related tasks like exercise, deep breathe or drink more water.

It is entertaining to eavesdrop in on is a group of friends or a married couple comparing their Fitbit daily step count. For we get a little squirt of endorphin from reaching 10,000 steps in a day or having just a few more steps than our spouse. We are a competitive species that need the motivation of simple rewards. Health apps and devices provide both, while encouraging a hands-on, take control approach to our health. Whether it is the number of steps that we walk, the amount of exercise that we accomplished, the miles that we run or bike, our heart rate, blood pressure or blood sugar, these tech devices make us more in charge of our own health. SPUN can encourage the development of more such devices by making it easy for a smart device designer to place their data into the system.

To further encourage patients to be masters of their own health, all our medical systems should be simple, open and inviting. It should not feel like working with the Internal Revenue Service (Apologies to my best friend, Bob, who works for the IRS.) or the cable company, which is how it feels way too often, today. Although medical systems, whether they are hospitals, medical offices or clinics, by their very nature must be very large and complex, they can be recreated to feel small and be easy to navigate. Do you want proof? Remember, our description of Amazon from the start of this chapter? If that company, one of the largest in the world, can make shopping online feel like a simple and fun experience, the same thing can happen in healthcare.

How do we make our medical practices, offices, clinics and

hospitals seem smaller? The answer is to encourage our providers to integrate and be bigger. I know it first sounds oxymoronic, but it is not. I hear your objections. First, you may say such integrations exists. True, there are growing numbers of and increased sized healthcare systems. Large hospitals buy or merge with smaller ones, only to be later swallowed by even larger ones. Hospitals also buy physician practices and create networks within them. Such trends, though, are merely mergers and acquisitions. They are odd collections with lots of pieces that do not fit together. They are like that junk drawer in your kitchen. They may be in the same place, but it does not mean they belong or fit together. For example, a group of hospitals may share the same paint color on their walls and logo on their stationary, but a typical patient's care takes place at just one facility. A group of hospital practices in a network may share the same boss but act independently of each other like that strange collection of stores at the same mall. For today, the purpose of these healthcare systems is just financial. It is so each can make more money as part of a group than it would on its own. It is not for the betterment of healthcare.

Another reason that the pieces of a healthcare network do not work together is the Stark Law. Like many things in American medicine, it is a regulation that was passed with good intention. However, it has caused more headaches than problems that it has solved and has long outlived its usefulness. The law is named after Pete Stark, a Democratic United States congressman from California, who wrote the bill which passed in its initial form in 1989. The real name of the law is the Ethics in Patient Referrals Act. The basis of the law is it prohibits physicians from referring to themselves. That is, profiting from sending patients for medical services where they have a financial interest in the business. For example, a doctor cannot send a physician to a laboratory if she owned part of it. Or an orthopedic surgeon cannot refer a patient to a physician therapy entity that he had a financial interest in. On paper, the Stark Law makes sense. It should help reduce medical costs from preventing physicians from referring patients for medical service they do not need just because they would make money from it. The law, since 1989, has undergone many modifications and has evolved into a complex web of regulations that include many different situations and exceptions.

Today, the Stark Law inhibits a health group from working together as a cohesive organization. For example, let us pretend that Dr. Joe is a family physician and Dr. Sally is a general surgeon. They both work for the same health system. Dr. Joe has a patient with stones in her gallbladder that requires surgery. Is it illegal for Dr. Joe to send that patient to Dr. Sally since he would indirectly profit from the referral of the patient to her since they both work for the same system? Questions like these keep health administrators up at night and help to employ many lawyers.

How can we create integrated healthcare systems? My proposal is called a healthweb. I call it a web because although the connections between the medical providers seem tiny, together they create a strong, unified and useful pattern. Plus, most of these connections depends on the internet. Get it? The world wide web? Healthwebs will be a group of medical providers from different areas of medicine working together to deliver a complete package of health services.

Healthwebs will vary in scope. There may be a healthweb formed from a group of dentists. They are organized include the dental specialties of oral surgery, orthodontia, periodontal care and endodontics, pediatric dentistry, dental pathology and dental radiology. The dental healthweb delivers total tooth care for a community. There may be a healthweb for eye care that consists of an integrated group of ophthalmologists, cornea, retina, glaucoma, plastics and neuro subspecialists, along with optometrists, opticians and eyeglass and lens facilities. At the other end of the spectrum, there may be a group of hospitals along with practitioners of all the medical specialties and subspecialties that provide from soup to nuts total healthcare for a region. Healthwebs need not be under the same corporate house or financial roof. They could be no different than a group of trades working together to build a house or a group of venders selling their wares under the Amazon or eBay banner.

Healthwebs will formalize and strengthen the bonds that today we see as just referral patterns. Medical practitioners like to make referrals to specific specialists when their patient needs care outside their expertise. Referral patterns develop for one main reason. It is not because practitioners get a financial kickback from a referral. It is not because some sort of cynical quid quo pro develops that if I send you ten patients, you will send back to me ten other patients. It is not because the referred specialist will cover up the referring doctor's errors in medical judgment. It is not because the referral group all golf together on Wednesday afternoons. It is simply because they like working with each other. They think alike. They have the same medical philosophies. And that is a good thing. It is a neat watching two practitioners of a referral pattern meet in a hospital hallway. They greet each other like long lost friends. You cannot help seeing the look of mutual professional admiration in their eyes. The advantage for us as patients for encouraging such connections is obvious. We get more consistent and more integrated care if all our medical care providers think alike and get along with each other.

Healthwebs will be much more than just consistent referral patterns. The various practices of a healthweb, even if they are corporately and financially independent of one another, will work together as one. They will share the same patient schedules. That is, they can book patients in each other's practices. They will share the same medical records, making the flow of information between practices easier for both providers and patients. These will be a piece of cake with the setup of our

SPUN EMR. They will share the same geography. That is, they may work in each other's offices or in the same building. Or at least, be close enough to each other for a patient to travel from one to another without much hassle.

Have you ever noticed that new car dealers seem to cluster together in the same location? That it is not unusual to see a Chevrolet, Ford, Nissan, BMW, Toyota and Honda dealer all lined up in a row on the same highway, even though they are completely separate dealerships? The same phenomenon happens in medicine. Medical practices cluster together. Commonly, they surround regional hospitals or occupy the same suburban office parks. Future healthwebs can take advantage of this natural clustering as they develop.

Let me give you some examples of how a future healthweb would work for you. You wake one morning with an awful toothache. Using your SPUN health app on your phone, you schedule an appointment that morning, with your dentist, Dr. Jennifer. She exams your painful tooth and takes an X-ray in her single practitioner dental practice office. Dr. Jennifer informs you that you need a root canal. She is part of a dental healthweb, called "Pearly Whites," and works with a Dr. Matt, who is endodontist. Drs. Jennifer and Matt went to dental school together, have shared hundreds of dental patients, and have similar dental philosophies. And his office is just across the street from Dr. Jennifer's. Since you are in so much pain by now, you will agree to any treatment by anyone. You just want to feel better. As she is speaking to you, Dr. Jennifer is able to schedule an appointment for you with Dr. Matt in 45 minutes. You walk across the street, find his office and are pleasantly surprised the staff are waiting for you. There are no forms to fill out. They have all your medical information and even the dental X-ray, Dr. Jennifer took. After a short wait, you are seeing Dr. Matt. He puts you at ease about your root canal surgery which he can do right then and there for you. You develop an instant trust of him both because of Dr. Jennifer's referral and their similar personalities. He does the root canal for you and it goes well. As you leave, he schedules a follow up visit back with Dr. Jennifer. When you see her for follow up care, she has all the records from the procedure performed by Dr. Matt. She gives you a clean bill of dental health. You thank her for the great referral and you are happy to be part of the Pearly Whites dental healthweb.

Imagine this second scenario. You made as one of your New Year's resolutions to take better care of yourself. After all, you are getting up there in years and have fallen too far behind in your checkups and health screenings. You also are motivated by all the incentives that SPUN gives you for completing such screenings. On the other hand, you have been busy at work, and it has been so hard to take off for all the necessary tests and appointments. Therefore, you decide to try out the new Medi One Stop healthweb. You figure if your family doctor is part of it, it should be okay. It starts with you using to your SPUN health app on your new iPhone 12S. It calculates for you a long laundry list of health needs. Blood work, mammography, bone density screening, gynecologic examination, eye, skin and dental screenings. Then its artificial intelligence arranges for you all those appointments in just one day at Medi One Stop. And as an added bonus, they all are in the same building. You are excited that you can get all the poking and prodding completed in one day.

The day of your appointment is a whirlwind. But you are amazed as you progress through it, how your care flows together. That is, even with the extra detours you must make. It feels more like a long day at the mall, Christmas shopping, than a medical maintenance day because you are in constant motion. The only check-in you make is for your first appointment which having your bloodwork taken. After your blood is drawn, your SPUN health app beeps on your iPhone, directing you to the next stop, the radiology department. It even gives you a map and directions to find it inside the medical office building. Here, your mammography and bone density scan go off without a hitch. There is no waiting or rush. As soon as you are finished, again, there is another beep from the app on your cell phone. It is time to see the dermatologist. There are more directions and still no waiting. The doctor performs your skin screening. She even has time to remove a couple of moles that you have been worried about. Afterward, there is some free time before your next scheduled appointment. Through the SPUN app, Medi One Stop suggests that you take advantage of a complimentary dietary consult that they are offering. You do and get some valuable advice about the glycemia index of various carbohydrates, which is important for you since you are prediabetic. As you are tasting some of the free, healthy snacks they have prepared as samples, you get a beep that your optometrist is ready for you. Your eye examination is normal, except you need a stronger pair of glasses. Afterward, an optician helps you pick out a pair that is flattering for you and promises the glasses will be ready for you to take home by the end of the day. Your app beeps again. And off you go for your gynecologic checkup. During the exam, your gynecologist thinks she might feel a cyst on your right ovary. To be sure, she wants to order a pelvic ultrasound to get a better look. Instead of having to schedule the test at another time on another day and wait and worry, the Medi One Stop appointment computer does some more magic by pushing back your dental checkup 45 minutes, so you can have the test performed for you right away. You even have time to go to another "freebee." It is a class on stress management which you attend as you drink the 32 ounces of water for your bladder to be full enough for the study. With your bladder bursting and some helpful advice on home-work balance, it is time for your ultrasound. As the technician performs the study, you look at the confusing sonar picture of your insides, wondering if you have cancer. Instead of waiting a week or more to hear the results, she has her findings confirmed by an offsite radiologist, right then and there. She even discusses them with your gynecologist. Great news! The study is completely normal. No cyst. No cancer. Beep. Beep. The dental office is now ready for you. Again, the flow through the practice is like riding the Swiss railway system. Teeth cleaning. X-rays. A normal exam. And the usual reminder to floss more. Afterward, you have a half hour break before your final appointment. It is just enough time to squeeze in one final complementary service, a manicure. You deserve it. After all, you have done so much good both for your body and mind, today. As your nails dry, beep, beep. Time to consult with your family physician. He, of course, has all the results of your tests and examination that have been done that day. That includes the blood work, mammography and bone density studies that started the day. Because he is not spending all his time on a clunky electronic medical record system or tracking down all your health records, he *talks* with you. He is not rushing, and he is *listening*, too! You feel your concerns about your health are being fully addressed. He discusses with you that you have the early stages of osteoporosis, based on your bone study that you had performed, that morning. He educates you on why you have it (family history, that you are fair and thin), why it is important to treat (your risk for bone fracture is high) and options for treatment (You both agree that a generic form of the medication, Fosamax, is the best choice for you.). He says the first month's prescription will be filled and waiting for you when you check out, today and that your future prescriptions will arrive automatically by mail. There is no need to go to a pharmacy or even having to order it online. Oh! By the way, he informs you that your new glasses are ready, and they are at the checkout desk, too. Your health screening day ends with you feeling really good about yourself. You have a new resolve to eat better to lower your blood sugars, exercise more, follow the advice about balance in your life, and take your Fosamax. You see more clearly. Your teeth are clean. And finally, your fingernails look great, too!

Does this all sound like a pipedream to you? It should not be. After all, I am asking no more of the healthcare system than what my dog received at the veterinarian office. All it takes is a group of professionals willing to work together, some changes to the system and some really good software. If Amazon can make buying a new book, a power cord for your iPhone, a sweatshirt and frying pan feel like you are shopping at one store, then the possibility of creating an integrated health network like the Medi One Stop exists. After all, what is more important, a piece of cookware or your heart?

How can we get there from here? How can the future SPUN Healthcare System nurture the creation of healthwebs? By now, you know what my first answer will be. Universal electronic medical records. For yet again, we can see the beauty of a single cloud-based system. Medical information will flow seamlessly among distinct parts of our health care system, even if they are freestanding independent entities.

Second, we need modern logistical management medical software. What does that mean? Today, patients move through their healthcare much as they did for the last one hundred years ago. Take scheduling. It is done with just the thought of one task for one patient. Patients, themselves, must navigate through multiple systems if they need more than one appointment. That typically means disjointed appointments all over town at different times and different days, performed in a non-logical order. That, in turn, means patients miss much more time from work and the rest of their lives. We are a less efficient society than we could be. Think of all the cars we could build, computers we could design, children we could teach and legal cases we could defend with that time we now lose as a society. No wonder we worry so much about Germany, China and Japan getting ahead of us. But it means even more than that. The complexity of the process means we avoid taking the necessary steps to be healthy, making us a less healthy society than we could be.

I hear you, naysayers. You claim that the logistic problem of the universal coordination of patient care is just too complex. Nonsense. Recent history is full of examples of how various industries outside of medical care have conquered their logistic problems and therefore have conquered the world. For example, during the 1960s and 1970s, Toyota developed "just in time manufacturing" in Japan. This reduced production times and costs in making their cars. It enabled a small company from a war-torn country to overtake the American auto industry and lead the world in just a few decades. Stop for a moment and think of what it must take to buy thousands of parts from hundreds of suppliers to make dozens of different types of vehicles in manufacturing plants all over the world. Scheduling a patient all her medical appointments on a single day should be a snap by comparison. Another business sector that has devised remarkable logistic results is the shipping industry. Think about the carrier industry and companies like FedEx, UPS and the postal service. And imagine the "impossible" logistics required to move a letter or a package from any address in the world to another and with different classes or speeds of service and being able to do so at a reasonable price. Companies like eBay and Amazon would not exist if these companies did not provide the necessary infrastructure for it to happen. In a similar vein, by providing the logistical infrastructure for our healthcare system, SPUN can nurture the future creation of healthwebs.

One necessary step SPUN must take to encourage the formation of healthwebs is knocking down the legal and bureaucratic barriers to their formation. We must accept a certain amount of bigness in healthcare, so it can give us the littleness we crave. Today, we are not logical about what big entities we allow and what we do not. For example, we accept the existence of just a few huge cable and internet companies and cellular networks but still have Stark Laws that prevent a couple of medical providers from working with one another. Bigness can be good. By turning a bit of a blind eye to the development and growth of such companies as Apple, Amazon, Google, Facebook and Netflix, it has allowed the United States to lead the world in technology. Imagine what potential exists for healthcare in this country, if we let it happen to this even more important part of our economy.

In June 2018, the heads of three completely different industries, all outside of medicine, announced to the world a joint venture in healthcare. Involved were some of the most famous names in American business, today. They included: Jeffrey Bezos of Amazon, Warren Buffett of Berkshire Hathaway and Jamie Dimon of JP Morgan Bank. The purpose of their joint venture was the creation of a health system to bring down costs for their companies and their employees. Although vague as to the details, just imagine the potential these three leaders, their companies with their resources could bring to our healthcare system. Although many writers fear such concentration of power and control in medicine, I welcome the innovation and imagination such business titans can bring. Like Silicon Valley fostered a creative environment for the computer and information industries, SPUN can create a similar one for the health industry. Perhaps under the right conditions, the United States can lead the world in how healthcare is delivered in the same way it leads the world in the technology.

In this chapter, we have seen that individual medical providers must take responsibility for each of a patient's medical problems. Primary care physicians must have ownership of an individual's complete health program. Patients need to oversee their own health needs. Healthwebs must be created to provide centralized systems of healthcare delivery. Now, one final need. And at the top of the nation's organizational chart, the proposed

SPUN must take a true leadership role for healthcare in this country. It is not enough just for it to be the universal medical insurance system. It is not enough for it to be the final arbitrator of medical rules and regulations. It is not enough for it to be the issuer of medical licenses. It is not enough for it to be the developer and controller of a universal medical record and information system. It is not enough for it to be the nurturer of future healthwebs. SPUN needs to be the organization responsible for all health and medical care in the United States.

Today, there are dozens of individual federal departments that control different wedges of the healthcare pie. Add to that, all the state and local health departments that have their sliver of control. Each have their own tiny domain with its own rules and regulations. The problem is that often overlap and conflict with one another. For example, today's federal medical insurance plans, Medicare and Medicaid, come under the Department of Health and Human Services. But part of Medicare falls under the control of the Social Security Administration, and the individual states each have their own rule sets for how they run Medicaid. For retired military personnel, that falls under its own cabinet level department, the Department of Veterans Affairs. The Departments of Labor and the United States Treasury are involved in running the Affordable Care Act (or Obamacare). The Food and Drug Administration, which oversees the safety of our medications and the Center for Disease Control, the overseer of public health for the country, both are divisions of the Department of Health and Human Services. However, they act like independent health services, rather than being integrated into a larger organization.

Ironically and perhaps not by coincidence, our country's health infrastructure today is a lot like the medical care that we get. There are lots of specialists and subspecialists. Most do an excellent job of the part of the pie that they are concerned with. But there is no one in control. There is no generalist in charge.

For we do not have a centralized department that sets policy for one-fifth of our economy that is devoted to our health. SPUN will be that future department. It will set what our health agenda and priorities. Its mandate will be both simple and critical. To give our country's citizens the best health possible in the most cost-effective manner.

Peter Lynch, the famous mutual fund manager and investor guru, once said "Never invest in any idea you can't illustrate with a crayon." The same should be said for any organization's goals and ideals. SPUN, when setting out its health policies should follow this simple crayon rule. There should be societal health goals that are open, specific, have a goal date and be reviewed. These goals then should generate clear policies and programs. For example, there should be not the goal of "reducing childhood obesity." It is not that I want American children to be overweight, but such a goal is too vague. Instead, the goal should be that the percentage of American children and teenagers, under age 18, that are overweight or obese, defined by a BMI of great than 25 should be reduced by 5% by the year 2025. With this goal in mind, SPUN can create programs, such as influencing school lunches and taxes on junk food, that can help achieve that goal. Then, in 2025, SPUN can evaluate if it achieved that goal. If it did, it can set a new goal for 2030. If it did not, it can look at what policies and programs failed and why did they fail. There should be goals for all aspects of health and wellness. From screening for glaucoma to reducing suicide rates, all of it should be specifically defined.

There is something about committing a goal to paper and setting a date to it that is motivating. If you just say you are going to lose some weight, your diet probably will not last a week or even to until dinnertime. If you say you are going to lose ten pounds by the week of your cruise to Bermuda, that is much more likely to happen, and you will look great for your trip. What is true for us, individuals, is true for organizations, the government and society, as a whole. Those of us of a certain age remember when President Kennedy committed the country to the goal of landing a man on the moon and returning him safely by the end of the 1960s. And we did. That is why it is so important that we have defined health goals as a society and the power of all our country's health resources out to achieve these goals. Committing them to paper can make them happen.

By now, you are thinking, how can take that first step? How can we make all these fundamental changes to our healthcare that we have discussed in this book? How can we go about create a SPUN or similar system that will deliver to us the healthy society at a reasonable cost that we deserve? That is the subject of our last chapter.

11. HOW CAN WE CHANGE?

My father, Leo, could fix anything. One of my most vivid memories from childhood is that we never had a repairperson come to our house. Whether it was a plumbing, roofing, an electrical or automotive item, my dad could analysis the issue at hand of why it was broken and come up with a solution for its repair. Being an engineer by training, he had an instinct for what to do. Motivated by his role model, I try to be like my father in this regard. I like to do my own repairs. Not only do I save money (and being "thrifty"), I get a pride of accomplishment. Today, it is an order of magnitude easier for me that it was for my father in his day. For I have the internet. Not matter what the house or car problem, there is a YouTube video or Wiki How webpage that I can refer to for help.

It is not enough just to list the problems that our American healthcare system is facing today and come up with solutions for fixing them. We must create a blueprint, a Wiki How page, a YouTube video, on how to do it. For our country, today, is having a difficult time figuring out how to go about fixing its problems, even when the solutions are obvious. This is the purpose of the final chapter of this book on the SPUN National Health Insurance Plan. How we can make it happen.

The first step in this process is realizing that we have a serious problem of how we receive and how we pay for healthcare in the United States. Today, that just is not happening. To be willing to change, we must see our problems. We must overcome our denial. For denial is a powerful human emotion and defense mechanism. When I practiced medicine, I often would become frustrated when a patient whom I was taking care of could not see that they had a serious medical condition. Whether it was their obesity, their hypertension, their depression, their diabetes or a large and suspicious mole on their skin, a patient would not take the necessary steps to seek out treatment until often it was too late. Interestingly, chronic problems elicited the most denial. There was less of a problem, if the patient had something sudden and acute. Severe chest pain, a stroke or appendicitis almost always gets our attention right away.

The same processes of denial occur at the level of a society. Although we react quickly to sudden problems, we, too often, have group denial about serious, slow evolving ones. Our history is full of examples of how our country ignored serious, chronic concerns. Too often, it took something sudden and acute that was a slap across the face to wake us up. Fascism was an obvious and serious problem in Europe and Japan during the 1930s. But the United States and the rest of the world was in denial about it until Poland was invaded by Germany and Pearl Harbor bombed by Japan. Radical religious fundamentalists threatened the United States for decades, but we neglected the warning signs before the attacks on the World Trade Center in New York and the Pentagon on 9/11. There were many warning signs of a housing and financial crisis for years before the banking system melted down in the summer and fall of 2008. Today, it is still happening. We deny or do not take serious enough the threat of climate change from our dumping of carbon dioxide and other greenhouse gases into our atmosphere.

What are we in denial about the state of our healthcare system? As outlined earlier in this book and described by dozens of other writers, the United States pays far more per person for medical care, both on an absolute basis and as a percentage of our gross domestic product than any other country in the world. And we do not get what we pay for. For we have the worst health and worst healthcare when viewed as a population among all the wealthy nations of the world. To make matter worse, the problem keeps growing each year. Healthcare costs consumes more and more, as a percentage, of what we produce as a society and our health statistics remain poor to mediocre.

This is a chronic problem. We did not get here as a nation, overnight. I remember in 1975, when I was just a college student, I wrote a term paper on the unsustainable growing costs of medical care in the United States for a sociology class that I was taking at the time. Then healthcare was only 7% of the gross domestic product versus over 18%, what it is today. Over those years, much ink was spilled and later, many photons on computers sent, describing the same problem. Every president over those ensuing years, from Gerald Ford to Donald Trump, has proposed fixes, but very little has been accomplished. Like all chronic illnesses, we have a national sickness that we do not recognize because we have been unwell for so long.

The results of this national chronic illness are threefold. Because we spend too much on healthcare, there are lost opportunities to accomplish so many other things as a society. Second, we have fewer human resources because we are not as healthy as we could be. Finally, and most important of all, because our lives are shorter and sicker, there is less human wellbeing and happiness than there could have been.

I have proof that we do not recognize that we have a national crisis in healthcare. Table 26 is a list of what Americans perceive are the greatest problems facing the country, today. It is taken from a Gallop poll taken in July 2018. Notice that healthcare barely makes the list, coming in way down the list, at number 7.

Table 26. Gallop Poll of July 2018 of the Top Problems Facing the United States

Problem	% of Americans Answering Yes
Immigration	22%
Dissatisfaction with government/ Poor leadership	19%
Race relations/Racism	7%
Unifying the country	6%
Lack of respect for each other	6%
Economy in general	4%
Healthcare	3%
Ethics/Moral/Religious/Family decline	3%

How do we fix our denial? Just like we must do for our own personal healthcare, we must be our own agents of change. We must educate ourselves about the growing American healthcare crisis. We must understand what alternatives we have for this national sickness. We need politicians, business leaders, healthcare thinkers to speak out and educate us. We need leadership that is ready, willing and able to make a change. We, as citizens, need to seek out, elect and otherwise support such leaders. A few such leaders do exist, today. Bernie Sanders, when he ran for the Democratic nomination for the presidency, in 2016, made healthcare a central part of his platform. He proposed a Medicare Plan for all Americans. Part of his appeal and why he almost won the nomination was his ability to strike this chord with so many voters. It is not just politicians on the left that want to talk about the crisis in the American healthcare system. Republicans, such as Senators Lindsey Graham from South Carolina and Bill Cassidy from Louisiana, speak often on the subject.

This leads us to the second step that is needed to enact the SPUN Healthcare Plan or a similar one. We must realize that the crisis in American healthcare affects all of us, regardless of our political views, whether we are rich, poor or middle class, whether we are young or old, and whether we are healthy or sick. Earlier in this book, hopefully I convinced you that everyone will save money on their cost on healthcare under my proposed plan. That included individuals, families and businesses of all types.

Our proposed SPUN Plan has something in it for both conservatives and liberals. It is not news that we have become a polarized country. There are some political issues that are especially divisive, such as abortion rights for women, immigration reform and foreign trade policy. Unfortunately, healthcare has become one of them, too. The Affordable Care Act, Obamacare, has been at the center of a national, political debate because the left wants an expanded role of government while the right wants a more limited role. If we are ever going to move forward as a country, we must be able to make grand compromises on these devise issues. And the leadership in Congress must set the example for us by being the first to make them.

The SPUN Healthcare Plan was not created with such a grand compromise in mind. It is based on the facts of our healthcare crisis and such plain common-sense conclusions. However, its conclusions have certain appeal for both Democrats and Republicans. Liberals should like its big federal government takeover of healthcare from the private sector insurers. They should like the low out of pocket expenses. They should like the controls placed on pharmaceutical companies and other large medical corporations. On the other side of the aisle, conservatives should like its liability insurance reform. The maintenance of the private sector for delivery of healthcare should appeal to them. Finally, the removal of the burden of paying for private healthcare by businesses, large and small, will be removed. That will make large corporations more competitive in the world and encourage the startups of more small businesses.

The third step towards creating our SPUN Healthcare Plan is to understand we must make a dramatic change in the delivery of healthcare. Small incremental ones, such as Obamacare will not work. As the saying goes, we cannot stand both on the dock and the boat. American history is full of examples of when powerful laws were passed by Congress that shifted the direction in which our country was going that changed and influenced our country for the good. The Northwest Ordinance of 1787 set a mechanism for new states to be formed out of the territories of the country. These new states were equal with the old so as the United States grew, it was not setting us up as a ruling empire of the elite states. The Judiciary Act of 1789 made the Supreme Court the final arbiter of the Constitution. This established one of the most important checks and balances in how our government is run. The Posse Comitatus Act of 1879 created a clear separation between the military and law enforcement. Its effect is our country could not drift into a police state which is so common elsewhere in the world to this day. The Pure Food and Drug Act of 1906 set up protections for the food we eat and the medications that we take. It was the first of many consumer protections acts that are the government's attempts to keep its citizens safe. Think of how radical Social Security must have been, when it was first enacted in 1935. It was the first time that the federal government said it was going to provide a guaranteed safety net for its citizens, in this case, its elderly. No longer were we totally on our own or dependent on charity or family if we fell into hard times. The Fair Labor Standards Act of 1938 gave us powerful protections as workers. It established such concepts that we take for granted today as the forty-hour work week and guaranteed overtime pay. The Civil Rights Acts of 1964 and

1968 with the Voting Rights Act of 1965 were huge steps forward to fix the racial injustices that have been present in our country since its founding. We are a much different country because of each of these laws.

For in each case of these landmark acts of Congress, political leaders saw a growing, unsolved problem for American society and took bold action to correct it by legislation. We need such decisive action in healthcare to reform it, today. We need the SPUN Healthcare Plan or similar, sweeping laws to fix how medical care is delivered and paid for in the United States.

The final step to take to reform healthcare in the United States is the hardest one of all. It is fixing what is most holding the country back from meaningful change. That is, the power of lobbyists and special interests' groups in American politics. Nowhere is that power wielded more, today, than in healthcare. Table 27 is taken from opensecrets.org of the Center for Responsive Politics. It is a nonpartisan, independent nonprofit organization that tracks money in United States politics and its effect on elections and public policy. It lists what the top ten industries spent on political contributions and lobbying efforts from 1998 until 2017.

Table 27. Political Spending by Industry in the United States from 1998 to 2017

Rank	Industry	Total Spending
1	Pharmaceuticals and Health Products	$3,591,651,507
2	Insurance	$2,466,283,140
3	Electric Utilities	$2,215,143,140
4	Business Associations	$2,046,757,727
5	Electronic Manufacturing and Equipment	$2,041,224,344
6	Oil and Gas	$1,939,997,877
7	Miscellaneous Manufacturing & Distribution	$1,575,859,569
8	Education	$1,534,652,750
9	Hospitals and Nursing Homes	$1,477,806,500
10	Securities and Investment	$1,431,255,478

This table is shocking on many levels. It is amazing that political spending is in the realm of *billions* of dollars. Notice, too, that the drug and related manufacturers are the very top of the list as the biggest group of political spenders. Just as shocking is that three of the top ten are involved in healthcare: the pharmaceuticals, the insurance industry, at number two and hospitals at number nine. If you want to know why significant healthcare reform has not happened in the United States, despite the desperate need for it, this is the answer. Certain entrenched portions of today's system do not want change from the status quo. Remember that money is the answer is nine out of ten questions in life. Their money talks.

Perhaps, first, we need a reform of our political system, first. Or at least how special interest groups and their money have too much influence on the system. Or perhaps, there are enough of today's politicians, who despite the money they receive from the various healthcare industries, have both the courage and the foresight to change our present system.

Why is it so important? We can have our cake and eat it, too. We can cut medical care costs enough that we can accomplish so many other things as a society. Whether it is solving the problem of global warming, improving our educational systems, or going to Mars. We will have the resources to do so, just by spending the per capita amount on healthcare to the number two country in the world. Plus, we can be much healthier as a people. We can live longer, have less chronic conditions and be vaccinated at a higher rate. We should be treated at least as well as my dog in the process. And not worry about how we are going to pay for it. Being healthy as we can be is a fundamental right and as Americans will see it that way, sooner or later. Let us make it a lot sooner.

ABOUT THE AUTHOR

William Frangipane is a retired obstetrician-gynecologist who lives in suburban Philadelphia. After having the privilege of delivering over 5,200 babies in his career, he now enjoys teaching, writing on subjects that he is passionate about, riding his scooter, traveling the world and summers at the Jersey shore.

INDEX

credentialing process, 148,
240, 248

criminal law, 207

CT scans, 27, 28, 29, 30,
197, 218, 221, 230

DEA, 144

deductible, 39, 40

deep pockets, 213

defensive medicine, 217,
219, 220, 221, 222, 223,
225, 231, 232, 258

Democrats, 33, 312

dentists, 134, 141, 228, 253,
296

Department of Health and
Human Services, 305

Department of Veterans
Affairs, 305

diagnosis related group, 149

DiCaprio, Leonardo, 239

Dimon, Jamie, 304

Disney Land, 2, 5, 16, 29,
166, 176, 285

DRG, 149, 158, 159

Drug Enforcement Agency,
144

drug patent system, 92

E. coli, 203

eBay, 161, 297, 303

echocardiogram, 184

EKG, 198

electronic medical record
systems, 163, 180

Elixir, 199

Emergency Trauma Center,
84

EMR, 15, 135, 164, 171,
172, 175, 177, 179, 181,
182, 183, 187, 188, 189,
199, 200, 201, 202, 257,
276, 281, 294, 298

enterprise system, 226

EPO, 38, 39

ETC, 84

Exclusive Provider
Organizations, 38

Facebook, 135, 188, 304

Facetime, 132, 172

www.ingramcontent.com/pod-product-compliance
Lightning Source LLC
Chambersburg PA
CBHW051342280526

45784CB00007B/2777